Mometrix
TEST PREPARATION

# Certified Midwives

## Exam Secrets Study Guide

AF834647

# DEAR FUTURE EXAM SUCCESS STORY

First of all, **THANK YOU** for purchasing Mometrix study materials!

Second, congratulations! You are one of the few determined test-takers who are committed to doing whatever it takes to excel on your exam. **You have come to the right place.** We developed these study materials with one goal in mind: to deliver you the information you need in a format that's concise and easy to use.

In addition to optimizing your guide for the content of the test, we've outlined our recommended steps for breaking down the preparation process into small, attainable goals so you can make sure you stay on track.

We've also analyzed the entire test-taking process, identifying the most common pitfalls and showing how you can overcome them and be ready for any curveball the test throws you.

Standardized testing is one of the biggest obstacles on your road to success, which only increases the importance of doing well in the high-pressure, high-stakes environment of test day. Your results on this test could have a significant impact on your future, and this guide provides the information and practical advice to help you achieve your full potential on test day.

**Your success is our success**

**We would love to hear from you!** If you would like to share the story of your exam success or if you have any questions or comments in regard to our products, please contact us at **800-673-8175** or **support@mometrix.com**.

Thanks again for your business and we wish you continued success!

Sincerely,
The Mometrix Test Preparation Team




Written and edited by the Mometrix Exam Secrets Test Prep Team
Printed in the United States of America

# TABLE OF CONTENTS

# Introduction

**Thank you for purchasing this resource**! You have made the choice to prepare yourself for a test that could have a huge impact on your future, and this guide is designed to help you be fully ready for test day. Obviously, it's important to have a solid understanding of the test material, but you also need to be prepared for the unique environment and stressors of the test, so that you can perform to the best of your abilities.

For this purpose, the first section that appears in this guide is the **Secret Keys**. We've devoted countless hours to meticulously researching what works and what doesn't, and we've boiled down our findings to the five most impactful steps you can take to improve your performance on the test. We start at the beginning with study planning and move through the preparation process, all the way to the testing strategies that will help you get the most out of what you know when you're finally sitting in front of the test.

We recommend that you start preparing for your test as far in advance as possible. However, if you've bought this guide as a last-minute study resource and only have a few days before your test, we recommend that you skip over the first two Secret Keys since they address a long-term study plan.

If you struggle with **test anxiety**, we strongly encourage you to check out our recommendations for how you can overcome it. Test anxiety is a formidable foe, but it can be beaten, and we want to make sure you have the tools you need to defeat it.

# Secret Key #1 – Plan Big, Study Small

There's a lot riding on your performance. If you want to ace this test, you're going to need to keep your skills sharp and the material fresh in your mind. You need a plan that lets you review everything you need to know while still fitting in your schedule. We'll break this strategy down into three categories.

## Information Organization

Start with the information you already have: the official test outline. From this, you can make a complete list of all the concepts you need to cover before the test. Organize these concepts into groups that can be studied together, and create a list of any related vocabulary you need to learn so you can brush up on any difficult terms. You'll want to keep this vocabulary list handy once you actually start studying since you may need to add to it along the way.

## Time Management

Once you have your set of study concepts, decide how to spread them out over the time you have left before the test. Break your study plan into small, clear goals so you have a manageable task for each day and know exactly what you're doing. Then just focus on one small step at a time. When you manage your time this way, you don't need to spend hours at a time studying. Studying a small block of content for a short period each day helps you retain information better and avoid stressing over how much you have left to do. You can relax knowing that you have a plan to cover everything in time. In order for this strategy to be effective though, you have to start studying early and stick to your schedule. Avoid the exhaustion and futility that comes from last-minute cramming!

## Study Environment

The environment you study in has a big impact on your learning. Studying in a coffee shop, while probably more enjoyable, is not likely to be as fruitful as studying in a quiet room. It's important to keep distractions to a minimum. You're only planning to study for a short block of time, so make the most of it. Don't pause to check your phone or get up to find a snack. It's also important to **avoid multitasking**. Research has consistently shown that multitasking will make your studying dramatically less effective. Your study area should also be comfortable and well-lit so you don't have the distraction of straining your eyes or sitting on an uncomfortable chair.

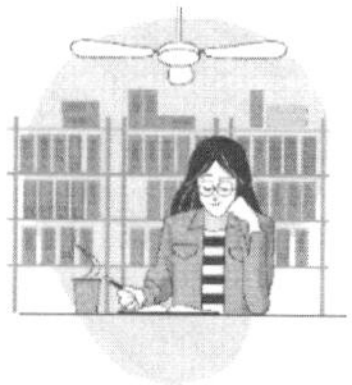

The time of day you study is also important. You want to be rested and alert. Don't wait until just before bedtime. Study when you'll be most likely to comprehend and remember. Even better, if you know what time of day your test will be, set that time aside for study. That way your brain will be used to working on that subject at that specific time and you'll have a better chance of recalling information.

Finally, it can be helpful to team up with others who are studying for the same test. Your actual studying should be done in as isolated an environment as possible, but the work of organizing the information and setting up the study plan can be divided up. In between study sessions, you can discuss with your teammates the concepts that you're all studying and quiz each other on the details. Just be sure that your teammates are as serious about the test as you are. If you find that your study time is being replaced with social time, you might need to find a new team.

# Secret Key #2 – Make Your Studying Count

You're devoting a lot of time and effort to preparing for this test, so you want to be absolutely certain it will pay off. This means doing more than just reading the content and hoping you can remember it on test day. It's important to make every minute of study count. There are two main areas you can focus on to make your studying count.

## Retention

It doesn't matter how much time you study if you can't remember the material. You need to make sure you are retaining the concepts. To check your retention of the information you're learning, try recalling it at later times with minimal prompting. Try carrying around flashcards and glance at one or two from time to time or ask a friend who's also studying for the test to quiz you.

To enhance your retention, look for ways to put the information into practice so that you can apply it rather than simply recalling it. If you're using the information in practical ways, it will be much easier to remember. Similarly, it helps to solidify a concept in your mind if you're not only reading it to yourself but also explaining it to someone else. Ask a friend to let you teach them about a concept you're a little shaky on (or speak aloud to an imaginary audience if necessary). As you try to summarize, define, give examples, and answer your friend's questions, you'll understand the concepts better and they will stay with you longer. Finally, step back for a big picture view and ask yourself how each piece of information fits with the whole subject. When you link the different concepts together and see them working together as a whole, it's easier to remember the individual components.

Finally, practice showing your work on any multi-step problems, even if you're just studying. Writing out each step you take to solve a problem will help solidify the process in your mind, and you'll be more likely to remember it during the test.

## Modality

*Modality* simply refers to the means or method by which you study. Choosing a study modality that fits your own individual learning style is crucial. No two people learn best in exactly the same way, so it's important to know your strengths and use them to your advantage.

For example, if you learn best by visualization, focus on visualizing a concept in your mind and draw an image or a diagram. Try color-coding your notes, illustrating them, or creating symbols that will trigger your mind to recall a learned concept. If you learn best by hearing or discussing information, find a study partner who learns the same way or read aloud to yourself. Think about how to put the information in your own words. Imagine that you are giving a lecture on the topic and record yourself so you can listen to it later.

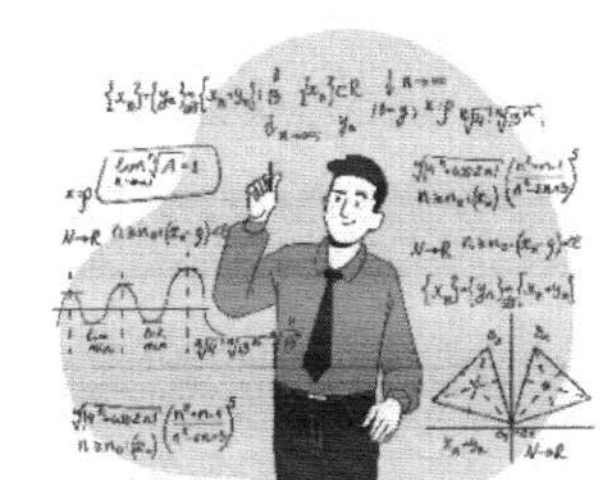

For any learning style, flashcards can be helpful. Organize the information so you can take advantage of spare moments to review. Underline key words or phrases. Use different colors for different categories. Mnemonic devices (such as creating a short list in which every item starts with the same letter) can also help with retention. Find what works best for you and use it to store the information in your mind most effectively and easily.

# Secret Key #3 – Practice the Right Way

Your success on test day depends not only on how many hours you put into preparing, but also on whether you prepared the right way. It's good to check along the way to see if your studying is paying off. One of the most effective ways to do this is by taking practice tests to evaluate your progress. Practice tests are useful because they show exactly where you need to improve. Every time you take a practice test, pay special attention to these three groups of questions:

- The questions you got wrong
- The questions you had to guess on, even if you guessed right
- The questions you found difficult or slow to work through

This will show you exactly what your weak areas are, and where you need to devote more study time. Ask yourself why each of these questions gave you trouble. Was it because you didn't understand the material? Was it because you didn't remember the vocabulary? Do you need more repetitions on this type of question to build speed and confidence? Dig into those questions and figure out how you can strengthen your weak areas as you go back to review the material.

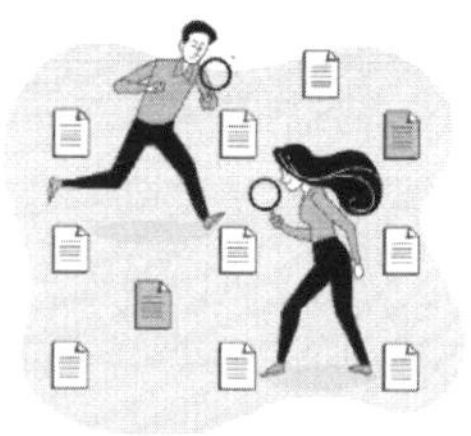

Additionally, many practice tests have a section explaining the answer choices. It can be tempting to read the explanation and think that you now have a good understanding of the concept. However, an explanation likely only covers part of the question's broader context. Even if the explanation makes perfect sense, **go back and investigate** every concept related to the question until you're positive you have a thorough understanding.

As you go along, keep in mind that the practice test is just that: practice. Memorizing these questions and answers will not be very helpful on the actual test because it is unlikely to have any of the same exact questions. If you only know the right answers to the sample questions, you won't be prepared for the real thing. **Study the concepts** until you understand them fully, and then you'll be able to answer any question that shows up on the test.

It's important to wait on the practice tests until you're ready. If you take a test on your first day of study, you may be overwhelmed by the amount of material covered and how much you need to learn. Work up to it gradually.

On test day, you'll need to be prepared for answering questions, managing your time, and using the test-taking strategies you've learned. It's a lot to balance, like a mental marathon that will have a big impact on your future. Like training for a marathon, you'll need to start slowly and work your way up. When test day arrives, you'll be ready.

Start with the strategies you've read in the first two Secret Keys—plan your course and study in the way that works best for you. If you have time, consider using multiple study resources to get different approaches to the same concepts. It can be helpful to see difficult concepts from more than one angle. Then find a good source for practice tests. Many times, the test website will suggest potential study resources or provide sample tests.

# Practice Test Strategy

If you're able to find at least three practice tests, we recommend this strategy:

### Untimed and Open-Book Practice

Take the first test with no time constraints and with your notes and study guide handy. Take your time and focus on applying the strategies you've learned.

### Timed and Open-Book Practice

Take the second practice test open-book as well, but set a timer and practice pacing yourself to finish in time.

### Timed and Closed-Book Practice

Take any other practice tests as if it were test day. Set a timer and put away your study materials. Sit at a table or desk in a quiet room, imagine yourself at the testing center, and answer questions as quickly and accurately as possible.

Keep repeating timed and closed-book tests on a regular basis until you run out of practice tests or it's time for the actual test. Your mind will be ready for the schedule and stress of test day, and you'll be able to focus on recalling the material you've learned.

# Secret Key #4 – Pace Yourself

Once you're fully prepared for the material on the test, your biggest challenge on test day will be managing your time. Just knowing that the clock is ticking can make you panic even if you have plenty of time left. Work on pacing yourself so you can build confidence against the time constraints of the exam. Pacing is a difficult skill to master, especially in a high-pressure environment, so **practice is vital**.

Set time expectations for your pace based on how much time is available. For example, if a section has 60 questions and the time limit is 30 minutes, you know you have to average 30 seconds or less per question in order to answer them all. Although 30 seconds is the hard limit, set 25 seconds per question as your goal, so you reserve extra time to spend on harder questions. When you budget extra time for the harder questions, you no longer have any reason to stress when those questions take longer to answer.

Don't let this time expectation distract you from working through the test at a calm, steady pace, but keep it in mind so you don't spend too much time on any one question. Recognize that taking extra time on one question you don't understand may keep you from answering two that you do understand later in the test. If your time limit for a question is up and you're still not sure of the answer, mark it and move on, and come back to it later if the time and the test format allow. If the testing format doesn't allow you to return to earlier questions, just make an educated guess; then put it out of your mind and move on.

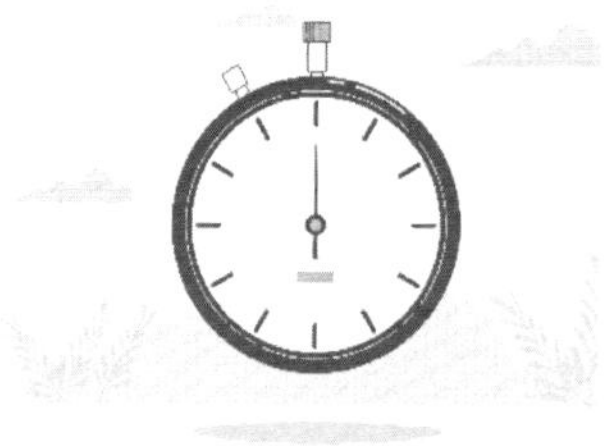

On the easier questions, be careful not to rush. It may seem wise to hurry through them so you have more time for the challenging ones, but it's not worth missing one if you know the concept and just didn't take the time to read the question fully. Work efficiently but make sure you understand the question and have looked at all of the answer choices, since more than one may seem right at first.

Even if you're paying attention to the time, you may find yourself a little behind at some point. You should speed up to get back on track, but do so wisely. Don't panic; just take a few seconds less on each question until you're caught up. Don't guess without thinking, but do look through the answer choices and eliminate any you know are wrong. If you can get down to two choices, it is often worthwhile to guess from those. Once you've chosen an answer, move on and don't dwell on any that you skipped or had to hurry through. If a question was taking too long, chances are it was one of the harder ones, so you weren't as likely to get it right anyway.

On the other hand, if you find yourself getting ahead of schedule, it may be beneficial to slow down a little. The more quickly you work, the more likely you are to make a careless mistake that will affect your score. You've budgeted time for each question, so don't be afraid to spend that time. Practice an efficient but careful pace to get the most out of the time you have.

# Secret Key #5 – Have a Plan for Guessing

When you're taking the test, you may find yourself stuck on a question. Some of the answer choices seem better than others, but you don't see the one answer choice that is obviously correct. What do you do?

The scenario described above is very common, yet most test takers have not effectively prepared for it. Developing and practicing a plan for guessing may be one of the single most effective uses of your time as you get ready for the exam.

In developing your plan for guessing, there are three questions to address:

- When should you start the guessing process?
- How should you narrow down the choices?
- Which answer should you choose?

## When to Start the Guessing Process

Unless your plan for guessing is to select C every time (which, despite its merits, is not what we recommend), you need to leave yourself enough time to apply your answer elimination strategies. Since you have a limited amount of time for each question, that means that if you're going to give yourself the best shot at guessing correctly, you have to decide quickly whether or not you will guess.

Of course, the best-case scenario is that you don't have to guess at all, so first, see if you can answer the question based on your knowledge of the subject and basic reasoning skills. Focus on the key words in the question and try to jog your memory of related topics. Give yourself a chance to bring the knowledge to mind, but once you realize that you don't have (or you can't access) the knowledge you need to answer the question, it's time to start the guessing process.

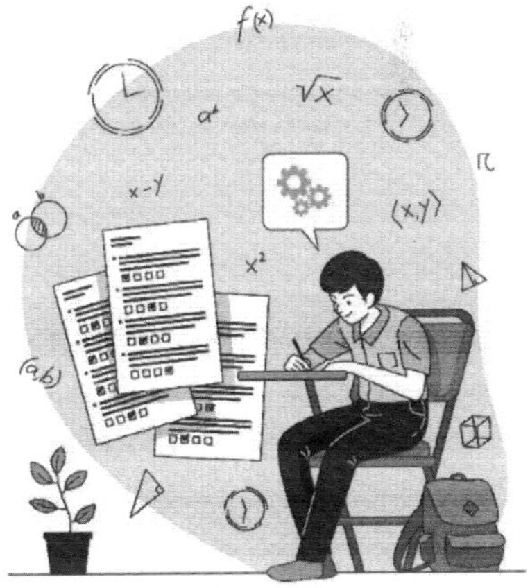

It's almost always better to start the guessing process too early than too late. It only takes a few seconds to remember something and answer the question from knowledge. Carefully eliminating wrong answer choices takes longer. Plus, going through the process of eliminating answer choices can actually help jog your memory.

**Summary**: Start the guessing process as soon as you decide that you can't answer the question based on your knowledge.

## How to Narrow Down the Choices

The next chapter in this book (**Test-Taking Strategies**) includes a wide range of strategies for how to approach questions and how to look for answer choices to eliminate. You will definitely want to read those carefully, practice them, and figure out which ones work best for you. Here though, we're going to address a mindset rather than a particular strategy.

Your odds of guessing an answer correctly depend on how many options you are choosing from.

| Number of options left | 5 | 4 | 3 | 2 | 1 |
|---|---|---|---|---|---|
| Odds of guessing correctly | 20% | 25% | 33% | 50% | 100% |

You can see from this chart just how valuable it is to be able to eliminate incorrect answers and make an educated guess, but there are two things that many test takers do that cause them to miss out on the benefits of guessing:

- Accidentally eliminating the correct answer
- Selecting an answer based on an impression

We'll look at the first one here, and the second one in the next section.

To avoid accidentally eliminating the correct answer, we recommend a thought exercise called **the $5 challenge**. In this challenge, you only eliminate an answer choice from contention if you are willing to bet $5 on it being wrong. Why $5? Five dollars is a small but not insignificant amount of money. It's an amount you could afford to lose but wouldn't want to throw away. And while losing $5 once might not hurt too much, doing it twenty times will set you back $100. In the same way, each small decision you make—eliminating a choice here, guessing on a question there—won't by itself impact your score very much, but when you put them all together, they can make a big difference. By holding each answer choice elimination decision to a higher standard, you can reduce the risk of accidentally eliminating the correct answer.

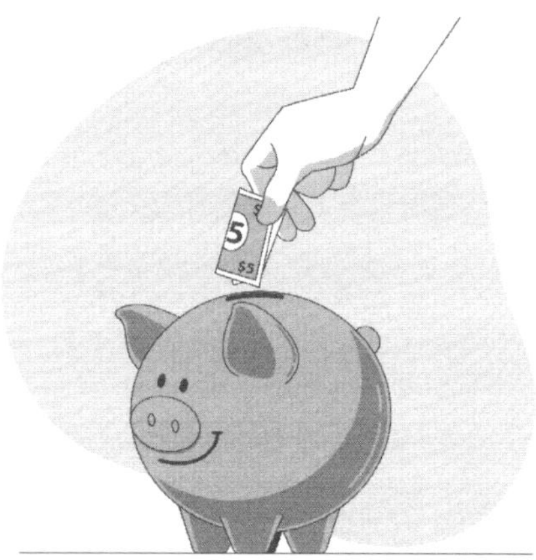

The $5 challenge can also be applied in a positive sense: If you are willing to bet $5 that an answer choice *is* correct, go ahead and mark it as correct.

**Summary**: Only eliminate an answer choice if you are willing to bet $5 that it is wrong.

## Which Answer to Choose

You're taking the test. You've run into a hard question and decided you'll have to guess. You've eliminated all the answer choices you're willing to bet $5 on. Now you have to pick an answer. Why do we even need to talk about this? Why can't you just pick whichever one you feel like when the time comes?

The answer to these questions is that if you don't come into the test with a plan, you'll rely on your impression to select an answer choice, and if you do that, you risk falling into a trap. The test writers know that everyone who takes their test will be guessing on some of the questions, so they intentionally write wrong answer choices to seem plausible. You still have to pick an answer though, and if the wrong answer choices are designed to look right, how can you ever be sure that you're not falling for their trap? The best solution we've found to this dilemma is to take the decision out of your hands entirely. Here is the process we recommend:

**Once you've eliminated any choices that you are confident (willing to bet $5) are wrong, select the first remaining choice as your answer.**

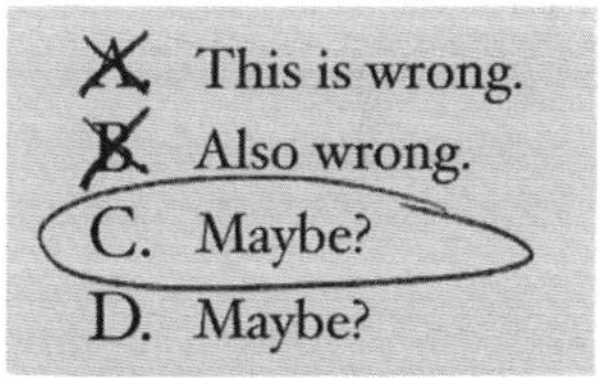


Whether you choose to select the first remaining choice, the second, or the last, the important thing is that you use some preselected standard. Using this approach guarantees that you will not be enticed into selecting an answer choice that looks right, because you are not basing your decision on how the answer choices look.

This is not meant to make you question your knowledge. Instead, it is to help you recognize the difference between your knowledge and your impressions. There's a huge difference between thinking an answer is right because of what you know, and thinking an answer is right because it looks or sounds like it should be right.

**Summary**: To ensure that your selection is appropriately random, make a predetermined selection from among all answer choices you have not eliminated.

# Test-Taking Strategies

This section contains a list of test-taking strategies that you may find helpful as you work through the test. By taking what you know and applying logical thought, you can maximize your chances of answering any question correctly!

It is very important to realize that every question is different and every person is different: no single strategy will work on every question, and no single strategy will work for every person. That's why we've included all of them here, so you can try them out and determine which ones work best for different types of questions and which ones work best for you.

## Question Strategies

### ✓ Read Carefully

Read the question and the answer choices carefully. Don't miss the question because you misread the terms. You have plenty of time to read each question thoroughly and make sure you understand what is being asked. Yet a happy medium must be attained, so don't waste too much time. You must read carefully and efficiently.

### ✓ Contextual Clues

Look for contextual clues. If the question includes a word you are not familiar with, look at the immediate context for some indication of what the word might mean. Contextual clues can often give you all the information you need to decipher the meaning of an unfamiliar word. Even if you can't determine the meaning, you may be able to narrow down the possibilities enough to make a solid guess at the answer to the question.

### ✓ Prefixes

If you're having trouble with a word in the question or answer choices, try dissecting it. Take advantage of every clue that the word might include. Prefixes can be a huge help. Usually, they allow you to determine a basic meaning. *Pre-* means before, *post-* means after, *pro-* is positive, *de-* is negative. From prefixes, you can get an idea of the general meaning of the word and try to put it into context.

### ✓ Hedge Words

Watch out for critical hedge words, such as *likely*, *may*, *can*, *often*, *almost*, *mostly*, *usually*, *generally*, *rarely*, and *sometimes*. Question writers insert these hedge phrases to cover every possibility. Often an answer choice will be wrong simply because it leaves no room for exception. Be on guard for answer choices that have definitive words such as *exactly* and *always*.

### ✓ Switchback Words

Stay alert for *switchbacks*. These are the words and phrases frequently used to alert you to shifts in thought. The most common switchback words are *but*, *although*, and *however*. Others include *nevertheless*, *on the other hand*, *even though*, *while*, *in spite of*, *despite*, and *regardless of*. Switchback words are important to catch because they can change the direction of the question or an answer choice.

### ✓ FACE VALUE

When in doubt, use common sense. Accept the situation in the problem at face value. Don't read too much into it. These problems will not require you to make wild assumptions. If you have to go beyond creativity and warp time or space in order to have an answer choice fit the question, then you should move on and consider the other answer choices. These are normal problems rooted in reality. The applicable relationship or explanation may not be readily apparent, but it is there for you to figure out. Use your common sense to interpret anything that isn't clear.

## Answer Choice Strategies

### ✓ ANSWER SELECTION

The most thorough way to pick an answer choice is to identify and eliminate wrong answers until only one is left, then confirm it is the correct answer. Sometimes an answer choice may immediately seem right, but be careful. The test writers will usually put more than one reasonable answer choice on each question, so take a second to read all of them and make sure that the other choices are not equally obvious. As long as you have time left, it is better to read every answer choice than to pick the first one that looks right without checking the others.

### ✓ ANSWER CHOICE FAMILIES

An answer choice family consists of two (in rare cases, three) answer choices that are very similar in construction and cannot all be true at the same time. If you see two answer choices that are direct opposites or parallels, one of them is usually the correct answer. For instance, if one answer choice says that quantity *x* increases and another either says that quantity *x* decreases (opposite) or says that quantity *y* increases (parallel), then those answer choices would fall into the same family. An answer choice that doesn't match the construction of the answer choice family is more likely to be incorrect. Most questions will not have answer choice families, but when they do appear, you should be prepared to recognize them.

### ✓ ELIMINATE ANSWERS

Eliminate answer choices as soon as you realize they are wrong, but make sure you consider all possibilities. If you are eliminating answer choices and realize that the last one you are left with is also wrong, don't panic. Start over and consider each choice again. There may be something you missed the first time that you will realize on the second pass.

### ✓ AVOID FACT TRAPS

Don't be distracted by an answer choice that is factually true but doesn't answer the question. You are looking for the choice that answers the question. Stay focused on what the question is asking for so you don't accidentally pick an answer that is true but incorrect. Always go back to the question and make sure the answer choice you've selected actually answers the question and is not merely a true statement.

### ✓ EXTREME STATEMENTS

In general, you should avoid answers that put forth extreme actions as standard practice or proclaim controversial ideas as established fact. An answer choice that states the "process should be used in certain situations, if…" is much more likely to be correct than one that states the "process should be discontinued completely." The first is a calm rational statement and doesn't even make a definitive, uncompromising stance, using a hedge word *if* to provide wiggle room, whereas the second choice is far more extreme.

### ⊘ Benchmark

As you read through the answer choices and you come across one that seems to answer the question well, mentally select that answer choice. This is not your final answer, but it's the one that will help you evaluate the other answer choices. The one that you selected is your benchmark or standard for judging each of the other answer choices. Every other answer choice must be compared to your benchmark. That choice is correct until proven otherwise by another answer choice beating it. If you find a better answer, then that one becomes your new benchmark. Once you've decided that no other choice answers the question as well as your benchmark, you have your final answer.

### ⊘ Predict the Answer

Before you even start looking at the answer choices, it is often best to try to predict the answer. When you come up with the answer on your own, it is easier to avoid distractions and traps because you will know exactly what to look for. The right answer choice is unlikely to be word-for-word what you came up with, but it should be a close match. Even if you are confident that you have the right answer, you should still take the time to read each option before moving on.

## General Strategies

### ⊘ Tough Questions

If you are stumped on a problem or it appears too hard or too difficult, don't waste time. Move on! Remember though, if you can quickly check for obviously incorrect answer choices, your chances of guessing correctly are greatly improved. Before you completely give up, at least try to knock out a couple of possible answers. Eliminate what you can and then guess at the remaining answer choices before moving on.

### ⊘ Check Your Work

Since you will probably not know every term listed and the answer to every question, it is important that you get credit for the ones that you do know. Don't miss any questions through careless mistakes. If at all possible, try to take a second to look back over your answer selection and make sure you've selected the correct answer choice and haven't made a costly careless mistake (such as marking an answer choice that you didn't mean to mark). This quick double check should more than pay for itself in caught mistakes for the time it costs.

### ⊘ Pace Yourself

It's easy to be overwhelmed when you're looking at a page full of questions; your mind is confused and full of random thoughts, and the clock is ticking down faster than you would like. Calm down and maintain the pace that you have set for yourself. Especially as you get down to the last few minutes of the test, don't let the small numbers on the clock make you panic. As long as you are on track by monitoring your pace, you are guaranteed to have time for each question.

### ⊘ Don't Rush

It is very easy to make errors when you are in a hurry. Maintaining a fast pace in answering questions is pointless if it makes you miss questions that you would have gotten right otherwise. Test writers like to include distracting information and wrong answers that seem right. Taking a little extra time to avoid careless mistakes can make all the difference in your test score. Find a pace that allows you to be confident in the answers that you select.

### ✓ KEEP MOVING

Panicking will not help you pass the test, so do your best to stay calm and keep moving. Taking deep breaths and going through the answer elimination steps you practiced can help to break through a stress barrier and keep your pace.

## Final Notes

The combination of a solid foundation of content knowledge and the confidence that comes from practicing your plan for applying that knowledge is the key to maximizing your performance on test day. As your foundation of content knowledge is built up and strengthened, you'll find that the strategies included in this chapter become more and more effective in helping you quickly sift through the distractions and traps of the test to isolate the correct answer.

Now that you're preparing to move forward into the test content chapters of this book, be sure to keep your goal in mind. As you read, think about how you will be able to apply this information on the test. If you've already seen sample questions for the test and you have an idea of the question format and style, try to come up with questions of your own that you can answer based on what you're reading. This will give you valuable practice applying your knowledge in the same ways you can expect to on test day.

**Good luck and good studying!**

# Midwifery Counseling, Education and Communication

## Prenatal Counseling

Many mothers have common fears regarding pregnancy and birth. You should both sympathize with her and help her resolve her own problems. The midwifery model of care defines counseling in terms of friendship and reassurance. Techniques such as mirroring, pacing, active listening, and positive reinforcement are all excellent ways to connect with the mother and work with her to resolve any issues. These techniques help identify the emotional tendencies of an individual and allow you to customize your communication. This personal approach is the opposite of the detachment of most medical models of care. This type of counseling should encourage the mother to accept the responsibility for her own fears and reactions. You should be aware of the boundaries of client privacy and pacing to prevent a codependent relationship and loss of objectivity.

## Pregnancy with IUD in Place

If a woman who has an IUD becomes pregnant there is a significant risk of intrauterine infection, placenta previa, premature labor, spontaneous abortion, and spontaneous septic abortion, and ectopic pregnancy. If the strings of the IUD are not observed at the cervical os or accessible in the cervical canal, use ultrasound to locate the position of the IUD. If the IUD cannot be found, it is possible it was expelled and arrangements for prenatal care or a therapeutic abortion can be made according to the woman's decision about maintaining the pregnancy. If the IUD is found but inaccessible for removal, a therapeutic abortion should be discussed since the risk of septic abortion in the second trimester is significant and life-threatening to the mother. The IUD should be removed in any case. Even if therapeutic abortion has been chosen, removal of the IUD decreases the risk of a spontaneous septic abortion prior to therapeutic abortion.

## Abortion, Spontaneous Abortion, and Threatened Abortion

Abortion is the termination of pregnancy with the expulsion of the products of conception prior to external fetal viability. This is an accepted definition to 20 weeks of gestation or 500 grams of fetal weight.

Spontaneous abortion (SAB): Commonly known as a miscarriage, this is an uninduced abortion, occurring naturally. The primary reason for this loss is genetic abnormality. Other causes are abnormal progesterone levels, thyroid conditions, uncontrolled diabetes, autoimmune disease, infection and uterine abnormalities.

Threatened abortion: This is a condition of vaginal bleeding during the first half of pregnancy. There may be cramping or lower backache. If both bleeding and pain are present, prognosis for the pregnancy is poor. A physical exam and evaluation of the serum BhCG and progesterone levels as well as ultrasound should be performed to determine the source of bleeding and treat it if possible.

## Missed, Habitual, Inevitable and Incomplete Abortion

Missed abortion: The fetus dies but the products of conception are not expelled for 2 or more weeks. There is a normal early pregnancy but without accompanying signs of pregnancy. There may be vaginal spotting or bleeding or lower abdominal or back pain at fetal death. The fundal height no longer increases and will decrease somewhat. Mammary changes will reverse. The woman will lose weight and no fetal heart tones will be present. Amenorrhea is present. An ultrasound should be obtained to confirm fetal death. There is a high possibility of DIC occurring. Refer to a physician.

Habitual abortion: This term is used if three or more consecutive pregnancies have terminated in spontaneous abortion. The woman should receive followup care throughout the grieving process, including counseling about contraception and sexual intercourse. Future pregnancy counseling should be given including genetic counseling, an endocrinology study, and examination to rule out developmental abnormalities of the genital tract.

Inevitable abortion: A spontaneous abortion (SAB) is highly likely to occur and cannot be stopped. Beyond bleeding and lower back or abdominal pain, there is also cervical dilation and/or rupture of the membranes. In the first trimester, the woman may be assisted by a physician to hasten the abortion with a suction D&C or she may wait for the abortion at home while monitoring for infection, heavy bleeding, or clots larger than 3 cm. Once she aborts she should contact the midwife. If there is a history of repeated SAB, the products of conception should be saved for genetic studies and confirmation of a complete abortion and intrauterine pregnancy.

Incomplete abortion: An SAB occurs without expelling the placenta along with the fetus. This may result in bleeding, possibly heavy, and infection, especially in the second trimester. Referral to the consulting physician is required to manage the infection and evacuate the retained placenta.

## Conception Timing with Contraceptives and Irregular Cycles

With birth control pills, the recommendation is to delay attempts to become pregnant until the first menstrual cycle has occurred signaling the likelihood that ovulation has resumed. If long term hormonal birth control has been used, such as Depo Provera or implants, it may take several months for regular cycles and ovulation to resume. A barrier method of birth control should be used until this occurs in order to accurately date the pregnancy. There is no issue of harm to the fetus by these birth control methods. Encourage the woman to keep a menstrual calendar.

If irregular cycles are an issue, basal body temperature charting or ovulation predictor kits are useful since predicting ovulation based on menses and subsequently dating the pregnancy are difficult in this case. If, after 12 months of unprotected sex, pregnancy has not occurred, referral to a fertility specialist may be in order.

## Birth Environment

The birth environment must be conducive to a relaxed labor. If you find this is not the case, you should assist the mother in making it so. Tell any family or friends the birth may be some time away. Only the birth team should be left and should sent elsewhere to give the mother some time alone or asked to cook for after the birth if needed. Once active labor has begun, you can ensure the mother has the setting needed to labor effectively. This may mean complete privacy, even from the birth attendant, and low light. You should not disturb her and should make certain others do the same. The partner may feel the need to assist; if so, the parents should be left alone to work things out and any interruptions should be minimal. Give plenty of warning and allow them to dictate when someone can enter the area.

## Birthing Centers and Home Births

A birthing center has many advantages of both a hospital and a home birth:

- The care focuses on natural childbirth
- The mother is allowed to make most of the decisions in her care

- Some medical intervention can be done if needed
- Transport is readily accomplished if attached to a hospital

Home birth advantages:

- The mother remains in a relaxing and familiar place
- Very little intervention is planned
- The birth is allowed to occur at its own pace

Home birth disadvantages:

- Emergency intervention can be delayed by transport if the hospital is not close by.
- Homebirth requires more of a commitment to self-reliance which may alarm a mother worried about the availability of medical care outside of the home birth attendant's purview, such as anesthesia, medical pain relief and other services available only through a medical center.

## Hospital Birth

The advantages of a hospital birth are:

- Quick access to emergency care during birth
- Availability of a "birthing room" as opposed to a "hospital room"
- Access to educational opportunities about childbirth and childcare
- Access to a number of caregivers and healthcare workers such as trained anesthesiologists to administer any desired medications or meet other needs

The disadvantages are that of a "managed birth" in which:

- The hospital staff may take responsibility for decision making away from the mother
- The same room may not be used for the entire process of labor, delivery and recovery
- The hospital may feel uncomfortable to the mother
- A mother with a normal birth and healthy baby must then go home shortly afterwards, without allowing time to adjust to or recover from the birth

## Considerations Regarding a Home Birth

Parents should discuss several factors before determining whether to have a home birth, above and beyond any pre-existing medical risks that may rule out a home birth from the beginning. The following issues can be discussed privately before meeting with you again:

- the reasons and perceived benefits for having the baby at home
- the perception of your duties
- the possible reactions to a hospital birth if one is required due to complications
- an enumeration of the risks and complications of birth that are known to the parents
- how any permanent disability or death of mother or baby will affect the parents

The answers to these issues may illuminate any incompatibilities with your style of practice and the parent's commitment to a home birth. Any reluctance on the part of the mother to discuss these issues is likely an indication of lack of commitment to a home birth.

## Preexisting Conditions Precluding At-Home Births

Certain conditions, which should be made apparent when a medical history is taken, preclude an at-home birth as each can create serious consequences for the mother, the baby or both.

- pre-existing diabetes or hypertension, thyroid disease (hyperthyroidism), chronic lung disease.
- severe asthma, epilepsy.
- clotting disorder, congenital heart disease, kidney disease.

Conditions occurring due to pregnancy contraindicating home births:

- Rh negative mother with antibodies.
- severe anemia that does not respond to treatment.
- acute viral infection such as rubella, cytomegalovirus, toxoplasmosis, chicken pox and herpes.

Other conditions precluding home births:

- unresolved sexually transmitted disease.
- malnourishment.
- drug addiction or uses alcohol moderately to frequently.
- smoking.

It is essential to have the consultation of peers or medical backup and availability of a comprehensive medical text to evaluate issues in the history.

## Contraindications to Home Birth

In some instances, there is no contraindication to a home birth, only the realization that the relationship between an you and a pregnant woman or her partner may not feel comfortable. Simply refer the mother to another midwife. In other situations, problems may not be evident until the first visit. This can include a contracted or abnormal pelvis, essential hypertension or extreme obesity. Psychological reasons play a role. There may be indications of irresponsibility, hostile reactions to suggestions for improved health, or rigidity in thinking processes. Smoking, drinking, or drug use that is not adjusted or eliminated in favor of the pregnancy or a poor diet may also be signs of unwillingness to adapt to pregnancy or work with you. If other behaviors or conditions become apparent that make you uncertain of the advisability of a home birth, consult experienced peers for assistance.

## Participants Besides the Midwife

The participants should continuously commit to any plans of care made for a home birth. All should be counseled regarding their responsibilities to maintain communication with the midwife including any life changes. Everyone involved must avail themselves of the reading material and educational classes that will assist them in a homebirth. Preparation must be made for breastfeeding, payment of any related fees, and relaying insurance information. Siblings and other participants must be educated about the experience to come and their responsibilities in it. All baby clothing, supplies and equipment must be obtained over the course of the pregnancy. Arrangements for other issues such as pet care and visits to care providers must be made and followed. Any supplies needed for emergency transport must be ready, including fuel for the transport car and a sure route to the hospital.

### Partner and Sibling Preparation for Participating

The mother's partner may need time to determine his or her role in the birth, or may be completely ready and willing to do whatever is needed or wanted. For some couples the act of the partner "catching" the baby is the most cherished wish of the pregnancy. You are responsible for ensuring the partner's education with appropriate reading materials, discussing the birth process, and depicting the sensual side of it. Use a model pelvis and doll for practice ahead of the actual birth. You must ensure the partner understands the emotional needs of the mother and to take all cues from the mother regarding the process.

Give siblings age appropriate books and show videos of the birthing process to give them a sense of what to expect. An adult companion for the sibling(s) should be present at the time of birth to care for them in the event they are overwhelmed by the birth.

### Preparation List for a Home Birth

The birth family should gather items specified by the midwife by 36 weeks. Supplies include:

- plastic covers to protect furniture and floors from blood and body fluids
- extra pillows
- nutrition for the mother during labor
- clean towels and washcloths
- antiseptic solution
- flashlight
- mirror
- bulb syringe
- 2-quart bowl
- heating pad
- thermometer
- measuring tape
- newborn receiving and clothing supplies
- squeeze bottle
- pads and underpads
- underwear
- alcohol and cotton balls
- large garbage bags
- Ziploc freezer bags
- hydrogen peroxide for blood stains
- emergency plan
- a list of phone numbers to be posted by the phone and in the mother's chart

In case of transport be sure to fuel the car; test the route to the hospital; complete and chart hospital admission forms. The home should be reasonably clean and all participants educated for the arrival of the new family member.

## HIPAA

A midwife legally:

- Must maintain the privacy of the client's healthcare information
- Must provide clients with written notice about privacy policies and practices, and the client's rights regarding personal information

- May use the client's information for treatment, payment, healthcare operations, to inform others in emergency treatment, when required by law, and if there is reasonable suspicion of abuse or neglect

The mother legally:

- Must consent to disclosing information to family and friends, for marketing services, or for any other purpose
- May revoke consent at any time
- Has the right to copies of her own healthcare information and a list of times when the midwife has disclosed the information for purposes other than treatment, payment or healthcare operations
- Has a right to ask for alternative methods of communication to maintain confidentiality and/or to ask the midwife, in writing, to amend her privacy practice
- May ask questions at any time about the practices
- Any complaints can be made to the midwife and to the U.S. Department of Health and Human Services

## Informed Consent

An informed consent document should be reviewed and signed by the midwife and the mother at the beginning of their relationship. It details the essential issues about a home or birth center birth. It should include:

- the advantages and disadvantages of the decision to be attended by a midwife
- the qualifications of the midwife
- the mother's consent to examination and treatment
- a summary of complications risked in childbirth
- a definition of common terms used during the pregnancy and birth
- details of the emergency equipment provided by the midwife and/or the birthing center
- an agreement to any hospital transfer recommended by the professional judgment and at the discretion of the midwife

An informed consent should open discussions between the midwife and mother regarding the important issues of home childbirth without creating an adversarial or fearful atmosphere. It should be a springboard, not a substitute, for a nurturing, trusting relationship between mother and midwife.

## Midwife Care

Midwives are often involved with their clients from the early part of pregnancy and offer continuous prenatal care. This affords them a chance to know their client exceptionally well and to intuit how the birth will go. Midwives tend to do extensive prenatal assessments which results in a more relaxed and predictable birth. Midwives see mothers as unique individuals who all have different needs during their pregnancy. This gives the midwife the information to assist each mother with the best practices for that mother. This also gives an advantage to the midwife at the time of labor and delivery. By knowing the mother so well, the midwife can more reliably tell whether all is going as it should, more so than if she was unfamiliar with the mother.

## Estranged Couples

You must assert your role as practitioner for the mother. You should not get caught up in the couple's problems. They may need referral to a specialist for counseling. They must be advised of the consequences to the birth if they are still indecisive about their relationship. It is to be hoped that the decision to remain together or to part will come early enough in the pregnancy to stabilize the mother's life. The mother must feel supported by her labor partner and may elect another in the life partner's place if support is lacking. If the life partner will be taking part, you should do everything to facilitate involvement. The mother should be counseled as a single mother in the event the partnership dissolves. This is also true of a mother presenting with a new partner. The couple may not truly be prepared to be parents together even with appropriate counseling.

## Pregnancy and Single Motherhood

A single mother who chooses to give birth at home needs the self confidence and self-esteem to overcome the lack of a birth partner. Any concerns she has regarding parenting can be allayed by stressing her positive traits and skills. Plans should be discussed for baby care for the first few weeks post-partum, as well as any fears of the birth itself, sexuality during pregnancy and after birth, and future hopes for relationships as they are expressed by the mother. Each mother must be approached regarding these issues in accordance with their unique styles of intellectual, emotional and spiritual behavior. Development of depression should be noted. The mother's social life and emotional outlets should be considered; however, the midwife has a responsibility to other clients and should not allow a mother to become dependent on her for continuous emotional support.

## Psychological Screening Out

Psychological screening out occurs when a client has emotional issues that preclude the probability of a successful home birth outcome. Before deciding to withdraw from the case, discuss the situation with the mother's backup physician so he or she understands any problems that may occur during the birth process. Also discuss the situation with midwife peers to avoid rumors and learn more regarding this type of client. Refer the mother to a recommended care giver who is more able to handle her case. Be firm with the decision to screen out. Avoid the temptation to accept the case later if the situation becomes better. It may not be due to improvement in the mother's basic issue. The decision to screen out will not allow the type of involvement you want but the alternative at best may be an unhappy birth situation and at worst a malpractice proceeding.

## Upsetting Information

When given the time to plan, you should determine the best way to give the news to each individual. Enough time should be allotted for the mother to absorb the information and ask questions if desired. Any other person or group the mother wants there should be brought in. All of the information regarding any problematic report should be readily available and the main points determined. Above all, honesty is required. No part of the information should be withheld. In addition, all the support you can give should be offered including personal time with the mother as well as referrals to any support groups or specialists. The news should be given as clearly and as simply as possible. The parents should be given time alone in a private room of your practice unless they wish to leave.

## Advocating for the Mother

Your primary role is one of education and support. If the opportunities are taken to educate the mother of her options and ensure they are clearly understood, the mother is then empowered to control her own pregnancy. Advocacy is defined as speaking for someone; in other words, ensuring that person's wishes are executed. In the medical establishment paternalism is still the norm and pregnancy is still treated as a medical issue. This leads health care workers to feel they must determine what is best no matter what the mother wants. Certainly, in medical emergencies, the medical staff must provide the correct care; however, during normal pregnancy and childbirth, the mother's choice should hold paramount. If she is not in a position to insist, you must advocate for her. This means the mother's wishes are known to you and you uphold the trust of the relationship by ensuring the wishes are followed.

## Early Labor

The mother should be well educated in the signs of early labor. The most obvious signs of impending labor are the "show", pink tinged vaginal mucus; spontaneous rupture of the membranes, commonly called the breaking of the water; or regular contractions, no more than 20 minutes apart. The mother should call you as soon as she thinks labor has started so you can make preparations. The mother should be taught the difference between "show" and excess bleeding that could indicate placental complications. Counseling about membrane rupture should include monitoring for bacterial infection, meconium passage, and the need to get rest while she is still able. When true contractions begin, it can be suggested that the mother get some light walking exercise, and she should be counseled to continue to eat and to sleep whenever possible.

## Sexual Abuse Survivor

A sexual abuse survivor may have a history of chronic conditions of the reproductive organs and menstrual cycle such as severe PMS, vaginal infections, eating disorders, and/or painful intercourse. If she has been previously pregnant there may be a history of hyperemesis gravidarium, premature labor, or repeated abortion. During pelvic exams she may react in one of two ways: she may show intense emotion to any exam of a reproductive part such as a breast exam or a speculum exam. Vaginismus may occur. Conversely, she may have a dissociative reaction where she may offer completely free access to her body but her mind and emotions are completely divorced from the proceedings. During the birth process, the loss of control may be especially abhorrent. Caesarian sections are prevalent and breastfeeding can be extremely difficult. Many of these reactions are also seen in victims of rape.

## Sexually Abused Mother

Women who have been sexually abused can be controlling, needy, or angry. In some instances, there may be no way to avoid accusations of wrongdoing as any action can become exaggerated in an abused person's mind. There are some guidelines for working with mothers with these issues. The midwife should not withdraw from any confrontation created by the mother. She should remain and actively listen. The mother's perceptions should be validated even if inaccurate or exaggerated. This diffuses anger and increases the chances of gaining and establishing trust. At that point, disagreements may be settled.

The midwife must also educate these mothers about their legal situation. Depending on the location, healthcare workers may be obligated by law to report evidence of violence to the authorities which can have an emotional impact on the mother. If the mother remains with the abuser, the midwife must determine a safe way of caring for her.

## Genetic Counseling

Genetic counseling should be recommended to those who:

- have an inherited disorder or birth defect.
- are pregnant or plan to become pregnant after the age of 35.
- have existing offspring with a birth defect or other inherited disorder.
- have lost babies in early infancy or had three or more miscarriages.
- may be exposed to hazardous materials.
- may have issues common to their ethnic group.

- are couples who are first cousins or other close blood relative.
- are pregnant and whose ultrasounds or blood tests indicate an increased risk for birth defects.

The family history and the parent's medical background are documented. Based upon this, blood tests, physical exams or amniocentesis may be recommended. The information is analyzed to explain the role of genetics in any condition discovered. Referral to a genetic counselor, resources, medical specialists, education specialists or support group is of enormous assistance in the parents' decision-making process.

## SMOKING

Smoking during pregnancy can increase the risk of prematurity, low birth weight, and stillbirth. At birth and throughout the first year, the infant has a higher risk of having respiratory problems, asthma, and otitis media. It has been shown that women who smoke 20 or more cigarettes are 15 times more likely to lose the infant to Sudden Infant Death Syndrome (SIDS) than a non-smoker. Other complications are spontaneous abortion, placental abruption, and placenta previa. Breastfeeding is still recommended even though nicotine is passed in breastmilk, as the benefits of breastmilk outweigh the risk of nicotine ingestion. Counsel the mother about these complications and urge her to stop smoking or to decrease the number of cigarettes she smokes each day. Refer her to a specialist or group that can help her stop. At this time, nicotine replacement therapy during pregnancy is controversial.

## DRUG ABUSE/USE DURING PREGNANCY

The effects of illegal drug use/abuse during pregnancy are many and varied. First and foremost, there is a high likelihood that the infant will go through withdrawal either during labor or after birth. The length of withdrawal depends upon the drug or drugs used by the mother as each drug has a different half-life. Additional problems include placental abruption, fetal distress during labor, intrauterine growth restriction and stillbirth. The mother is also less likely to obtain regular prenatal care or neonatal followup. She is unlikely to disclose her drug use to her medical care workers. Due to the typical lifestyle of a drug user, there is a greater risk of infectious disease such as Hepatitis B and C and/or HIV and the attendant complications of those diseases, as well as having poor housing, possibly other children with problems, and a lifestyle not conducive to raising a child.

## SOCIETAL PERCEPTION OF MOTHERHOOD

Society may see the birth of an infant as the culmination of a woman's reason for being. While there is no financial gain, her status is raised and her femininity is proven. However, if the mother herself feels less than completely ecstatic about motherhood and her baby, she is unlikely to admit it because she thinks that society would then see her as a "bad" mother. The emotional distress is internalized, creating stress and loss of sleep, which in turn erodes the ability to cope with the new lifestyle. In rare extremes, the mother may suffer severe psychological trauma and endanger herself or her children. With a mobile society, it is less likely the new mother has family available to help She becomes isolated and unsure of her success in her new role.

## PRECONCEPTION CARE FOR CHRONIC HEALTH ISSUES

Women who have epilepsy, chronic hypertension, psychoses, malaria and some other conditions are usually managing the illness using a medication that is teratogenic to a fetus. You must work with the client's physician who is treating the illness to try to find alternatives for the medications and to determine the risk to the fetus in the event the client has already conceived. No client should discontinue any prescribed treatment for such disorders without a physician's guidance. In addition to these conditions and the known teratogenic nature of many of the medications used to treat them, the teratogenicity of all medications taken during pregnancy must be assessed, whether the medication is prescription or over the counter (OTC). The risk/benefit ratio of medication use during pregnancy should be discussed prior to conception whenever possible.

## HPV

Human Papilloma Virus (HPV) is the most common sexually transmitted disease although it can also be contracted without sexual contact. It is possible for a mother to be unaware of the infection because there may be no outward signs of infection at all. HPV can be seen as condyloma accuminata, or visible genital warts, as well as flat lesions that are less visible. The warts can be treated topically but there is no cure for HPV. Some genotypes of HPV may be precursors to abnormal cell growth that can develop into cervical cancer. When HPV is diagnosed, it is recommended that pap smears be taken every 6 months to aid in early cancer diagnosis. HPV infection can be passed to the infant during birth. Genital warts may enlarge during pregnancy. Some treatments may harm the fetus in utero and must be avoided during pregnancy.

### Chlamydia

Chlamydia is a common Sexually Transmitted Disease (STD) in the United States second in incidence only to Human Papilloma Virus (HPV). Women are often asymptomatic but chlamydia can cause:

- Urinary tract infection
- Infection of the amniotic sac and fluid
- Premature labor or premature rupture of the membranes (PROM)
- Increased susceptibility to HIV
- 70% chance of fetal infection upon delivery
- Fetal conjunctivitis
- Fetal pneumonia

Gonorrhea is often seen in conjunction with chlamydia. If either one or both of these infections are present, both partners must be treated and must use barrier-type birth control until the infection is resolved. Tetracycline may not be used because it causes discoloration of the fetal tooth enamel. Erythromycin is the antibiotic of choice.

### Gonorrhea

Gonorrhea is a sexually transmitted disease. Infected women are often asymptomatic but can exhibit pain and burning upon urination, increase vaginal discharge or bleeding or spotting. Male partners often exhibit discharge and pain and burning upon urination.

Complications during pregnancy include:

- Chorioamnionitis
- Premature rupture of the membranes
- Preterm labor
- Fetal blindness if antibiotic drops are not instilled into the eyes within 2 hours of birth
- Fetal joint infection or sepsis

Gonorrhea is often seen in conjunction with Chlamydia. If either one or both of these infections are present, both partners must use barrier-type birth control until the infection is resolved.

## HEPATITIS C

Hepatitis C (HCV) is transmitted by blood and blood products and by sexual transmission. Symptoms of active infection are similar to Hepatitis B (nausea, vomiting, upper right quadrant abdominal pain, chills and fever), but 85% of cases become chronic. Transmission to the fetus occurs in about 5% of cases depending on the viral load of the mother's bloodstream but breast milk is not impacted. About 20% of hepatitis cases in the United States are HCV. There is no immunization for this virus. A mother who tests positive for HCV should be referred to her backup physician and also counseled that she may require liver function evaluation with blood tests and possibly a liver biopsy. Treatment for HCV includes injections of alpha interferon and oral ribavirin (an antiviral). However, ribavirin is a teratogenic drug and this treatment is contraindicated in pregnancy.

## HEPATITIS B

Hepatitis B (HBV) can be transmitted through blood and through body fluids such as semen, saliva, or vaginal secretions. It is highly contagious and mothers who are Hepatitis B Surface Antigen (HbsAG) positive are highly likely to transmit the virus to the baby. The baby can then become a carrier and may pass the virus to their own children. Babies born to HbsAG positive mothers must be immunized within 12 hours of birth to avert this problem. If immunized, the baby can then be breastfed by the mother. Mothers with active HBV infections should be hospitalized and all family members screened. Active infection is characterized by nausea, vomiting, upper right quadrant abdominal pain, chills and fever. An HBV carrier may be asymptomatic and will be positive for Hepatitis B Core Antibody (HbcAB).

## HIV SCREENING

All women should be screened for HIV, in particular those who have ever shared a needle or had unprotected sexual relations. Testing can be performed anonymously. The ELISA test is most commonly used but has a false positive rate of about 10%. A second positive test is required to reflex to Western Blot, a more specific test. An untreated seropositive mother has a 25% risk of passing the infection to the baby: 5-10% prenatally, 20% during labor and birth, and 5-15% during breastfeeding. The mother must be fully informed of all risks, both of treatment and non-treatment, and of related symptoms. The backup physician should be consulted regarding whether the midwife should continue primary care. Additionally, the midwife must define protocol for assisting anyone with a life-threatening, highly infectious disease since there is no immunization for HIV and, although Universal Precautions will be used, there is still a risk of infection to the health care worker.

## FEARS OF PREGNANCY COMPLICATIONS

Ask parents to tell you the worst of their fears regarding negative outcomes such as hospital transport or life threatening complications. This helps evaluate the parent's commitment to a home birth and also introduces the topic of complications and how they occur. It can then be emphasized that good prenatal care does much toward preventing many of the complications of labor and birth. This may impress upon them the importance of keeping appointments and informing you of any worrisome developments. Two of the most serious discussions are about hemorrhage and fetal distress. These topics should be discussed early in the pregnancy since there is no time to explain during such emergencies. The explanations should include possible causes of these issues, your procedures for handling them, your training, tools and techniques for stopping bleeding and resuscitating the baby.

## Grieving Process of a Lost Pregnancy

Both parents must be counseled regarding the effect the loss of a baby will have on them. Grieving for the loss of a pregnancy is the same as grieving any other loss of a loved one. Most people pass through certain stages as they grieve, not always in the same order as another person. The stages are:

- denial
- anger (at the self, the spouse, or God for letting it happen)
- guilt: (could it have been avoided by being more careful?)
- depression
- acceptance

Men and women grieve differently. Women are generally more expressive about their grief and will look for support. Men more often grieve in solitude. Men also have a tendency toward problem solving and fact gathering, choosing not to participate in a support setting. Memorializing the baby, no matter what stage the loss occurred can serve as a way to gain closure.

## Fetal Anomalies

### *Parental Support*

When a baby is born with anomalies, the parents will still bond with the baby, often only noticing the beauty of the other features. You should remain present until the anomaly is noted. If the parents seem to be in denial of the anomaly, it should be pointed out without extended discussion. If a severely deformed infant is rejected by the mother, you can encourage her to bond by helping her to see the perfect features the baby does have. You should stay in close contact with the parents for several months, assisting them by referring them to resources for information and support. The Internet is a valuable tool.

### *Assisting a Birth with Previously Unknown Fetal Anomalies*

The most common anomaly is a heart defect presenting as cyanosis and respiratory distress. Heart defects and spina bifida require immediate newborn transportation and pediatric consultation. Most other anomalies do not require immediate treatment but should be seen as soon as possible to determine the extent of the anomaly.

Fetal anomalies can be genetic or caused by viruses, chemicals, pharmaceuticals, radiation, or street drugs. If the anomalies are so severe that they are incompatible with life, follow the parents' lead regarding transport but you are obligated to give life support and call emergency services if the baby seems viable.

## History of Previous Abortion

The mother must be ready to discuss the abortion in order for you to obtain accurate information without causing her undue emotional distress. The method of abortion is important to note as each method holds risks for the future ability to become pregnant and to carry a baby to term. Dilation and curettage involves scraping of the endometrium which may cause scarring, creating a risk of interference with placental implantation. Suction is less damaging to the endometrial lining. A thorough discussion should be made of the decision to abort as well as the emotional impact of the abortion itself. Many women feel the same great sense of loss as women who have experienced repeated miscarriage.

### Female Reproductive System

The female reproductive system consists of the pelvic floor, vulva, vagina, uterus, Fallopian tubes, and ovaries. The pelvic floor supports the abdominal and pelvic organs. The muscles control urination and defecation and gives slight control to the passage of the fetus. It includes the perineal body: the muscle and tissue between the vagina and the rectum. The vulva includes all external genital organs: the mons pubis, labia majora, labia minora, clitoris, vestibule, urethral orifice, vaginal orifice, and Bartholin's glands. The vagina excretes menstrual flow, encloses the penis, receives sperm, and forms an opening for the fetus. Posterior to the vagina lays the pouch of Douglas, rectum and perineal body. Superiorly lies the uterus; and inferiorly lies the external genitalia. The uterus holds the fetus. The Fallopian tubes push the ovum toward the uterus, receive the sperm, and allow fertilization. The ovaries produce ova, estrogen and progesterone.

### Breast Self-Examination

Self breast examination and its importance should be taught at the time of the breast exam. Education should include an assessment of the knowledge already possessed by the mother and whether she performs self breast examination on a regular basis. If the mother does not know how to perform the exam, the following elements should be covered:

- why regular self-exams are important
- to perform the exam every month 24-48 hours after the end of a menstrual period
- positions in front of the mirror for visual inspection and what to look for
- the supine position with shoulder lifted on a pillow for palpation including exam with the arm raised and lowered
- proper palpation technique and what to look for
- what the normal structure is of the breast area

If the mother states she performs the self exam already, ask her to demonstrate it for you. If she does not or will not perform the exam, try to find out why.

### Kegel Exercises

Kegel exercises, also called pelvic floor exercises, help to strengthen the pelvic floor muscles and maintain urethral and anal sphincter function before and after birth. It also builds awareness of the muscles and the ability to manipulate them to ease some aspects of giving birth. Typically, the bladder is emptied. The pelvic floor muscles are tightened and held for about 10 seconds, then released for 10 seconds. The exercise is repeated up to 10 times. The exercises are performed three times a day. The proper performance of these exercises is important but difficult to discern. The thighs or abdomen may be tightened in error. Awareness of the various muscles within the peritoneal area must be taught in order to avoid these errors. One method of teaching the proper way of doing Kegels is to have the woman sit on the toilet, begin to urinate, and then stop the flow.

### Rubella Antibody Titer

The rubella antibody titer indicates the level of immunity that the mother has to German measles (Rubella). A titer greater than 1:10 indicates a prior infection or vaccination conferring immunity to rubella. An unusually high titer, greater than 1:64, may indicate a recent or current infection. Anything less than 1:10 is low and the mother may not have immunity. In this instance, the mother must be immunized after the current pregnancy and three months prior to becoming pregnant again. Vaccination while pregnant is contraindicated because the vaccine is a live attenuated virus that may impact the fetus. In the meantime, the mother must avoid infection since rubella infection during pregnancy can cause fetal cardiac defects, cataracts, and deafness in 20% of infants. It can also cause miscarriage, stillbirth, and fetal anomalies. Intrauterine and postnatal growth restriction may also occur.

### Chicken Pox

85-95% of expectant mothers are immune to chicken pox. However, 1 in 2000 non-immune women may develop chicken pox during pregnancy. If the infection occurs prior to 20 weeks gestation, there can be serious consequences to the fetus. The baby has a less than 1% chance of being born with congenital varicella syndrome. Defects include cataracts, chorioretinitis, limb hyperplasia, hydronephrosis, microcephaly, intellectual disability, dermatome lesions and cutaneous scars. If the infection is at the time of birth the baby can contract chicken pox infection and must be treated to keep the infection mild. Without treatment 30% of babies will die. A blood test can determine immunity and, if performed before pregnancy, the woman can be vaccinated and advised to wait a month prior to becoming pregnant. If a pregnant woman who is not immune comes into contact with an infected person, an injection of VZIG can prevent infection or lessen the severity, and is safe for both mother and baby.

### Toxoplasmosis

Toxoplasmosis is a protozoan infection. If contracted after the tenth week of gestation it can cause congenital anomalies, the most severe of which are:

- anencephaly
- hydrocephalus
- microcephaly
- intracranial calcifications

Many babies do not show symptoms at the time of birth. The condition can continue to cause symptoms throughout childhood such as seizures or intellectual disability. Toxoplasmosis can be contracted through raw or undercooked meat that has been infected, or by exposure to cat feces or contaminated soil. The best way to avoid it is to avoid eating raw or undercooked meat, especially pork, and to refrain from emptying a cat's litter box or coming into contact with a cat's feces in any other way. You should take a careful history in order to uncover any way in which the mother may be put at risk of this or other illnesses. Infection can be prevented through education and counseling.

### Parvovirus B19

Parvovirus is transmitted by respiratory secretion and percutaneous exposure to infected blood or blood products. It is a common virus in school aged children. If infection occurs during pregnancy, 20-30% of fetuses will become infected. Of those fetuses, some will develop aplastic anemia or nonimmune hydrops. In rare cases, the infection is fatal. Infection in the first half of pregnancy results in the most serious infections. If a pregnant woman is exposed, serum IgM and IgG should be tested for immunity. Negative results should trigger a repeat test three to four weeks later. With seroconversion the fetus must be monitored on a weekly basis for fetal hydrops, placentomegaly, and fetal growth restriction. Referral to a physician is advised.

### CMV

Cytomegalovirus (CMV) is part of the herpesvirus group. A majority of people in the United States have been infected with no long term issues. This virus, which is inactive once the primary infection is over, is usually transmitted to the fetus prior to birth. However, if the primary infection occurs during pregnancy, the fetus may be at risk. Thirty percent will become infected. Less than fifteen percent are symptomatic ranging from jaundice and moderate enlargement of the liver and spleen to fatality. Most will survive but many will develop such abnormalities as hearing loss, intellectual disability, and some blindness. Those who are asymptomatic may still develop some degree of these complications. The virus may not infect the infant until birth when genital secretions or breast milk may pass along the virus, but in these cases there is little to no illness demonstrated.

### Environmental Hazards to Pregnancy

Environmental hazards are found at home and in the workplace and can cause conditions from premature labor to fetal death. Hazards are chemicals, heavy metals, temperature issues, radiation, infectious agents, and stress.

Lead based paint is an environmental hazard that is a common public health issue. Lead exposure during pregnancy can cause miscarriage, low birth weight and developmental disorders. Lead exposure can also come from the workplace. Other environmental hazards include exposure to drugs such as cancer treatments, ethylene glycol ethers, and jobs that require heavy physical labor. Health care workers or animal workers are at particular risk of exposure to any number of infectious agents in the workplace. Most infections can be prevented by proper hand-washing or vaccination prior to pregnancy.

A thorough history reveals most of the hazards the mother is exposed to and you should discuss the consequences of exposure to her and her fetus and how problems can be prevented.

### Teratogenic Substances

A teratogenic substance is one that causes congenital defects in the unborn fetus. The Food and Drug Administration (FDA) maintains a list of categories sorting drugs according to their teratogenicity. Many are drugs; an example is thalidomide, which caused infants to be born with limb reductions. Maintaining access to this information is highly recommended for your reference. The type and severity of deformity may depend upon the timing of the exposure during gestation. A thorough history that includes any medications the woman is taking or handles should open a discussion of this issue and create awareness in the parents about examining all medications and other substances that are commonly taken or used in the home or at work. Ideally this discussion takes place prior to conception but in most cases must be addressed as soon as possible after conception.

### FDA Labeling Criteria

The FDA has five labeling categories for medications that may be used during pregnancy. These categories attempt to identify the risk to the fetus from specific drugs. The FDA categories and their definitions are as follows:

- **A**: Failure to demonstrate a risk to the fetus in the first trimester through human studies, risk of fetal harm remote.
- **B**: Animal studies show no risk to the fetus or do show risk but studies in pregnant women show no risk.
- **C**: Animal studies show the drug to be teratogenic to animal fetus, but no human studies or no animal or human studies performed.
- **D**: Positive evidence of teratogenicity but beneficial for certain reasons that may make drug use acceptable.
- **X**: Definite serious teratogen as demonstrated by fetal abnormalities found during studies or fetal risk demonstrated based on human experience, or both. Risk outweighs any benefit.

Decisions on the use of a specific drug should be made by the mother in conjunction with the midwife and the physician.

# General Healthcare Skills

## Accurate and Complete Record-Keeping

A medical chart is a legal document. The chart must contain all records of assessments, procedures, recommendations, discussions with the patient and other care providers, and all observations during any examination and during the birthing process in case of lawsuit. For legal defensibility the records must be written on lined paper, all notes must be continuous with only the midwife's initials and time/date to interrupt the flow. Leave no empty space, or partially or completely empty lines. Blank areas can invalidate an entire chart by creating the possibility of recording after the original time and date stamped. If information must be crossed out, a single line plus the midwife's initials, date and reason for cross-out must be written in. No information should be obliterated in any way. In some instances, the mother's initials may also be required, such as when she declines a recommended procedure or when stating understanding of the risks of a procedure. Accurate and complete charting is also helpful in establishing the midwife's professionalism.

## Universal Precautions

The Centers for Disease Control and Prevention have set out precautions to be followed by health care workers during interactions with all clients regardless of blood-borne infection status. These Universal Precautions are set out in a CDC document entitled "Recommendations for Prevention of HIV Transmission in Healthcare Settings". For midwives, the following precautions are relevant:

- Use barrier precautions (gloves, waterproof gowns or aprons, protective eyewear, and mouthpieces for resuscitation) to prevent skin and mucus membrane exposure to blood, amniotic fluid, vaginal secretions, seminal fluid, and breast milk.
- Use gloves for blood and culture collection, vaginal exams, assisting delivery, handling the newborn prior to its cleaning and handling soiled under-pads, clothing or bed linens.
- Immediately wash hands and skin if they become contaminated and consult a health care professional.
- Dispose of all used sharp instruments and needles in a puncture resistant container. Never recap or excessively handle such items.

## Herbs for Pregnancy Support

Herbal infusions are one method of ingesting herbs; one ounce of herb to one quart of boiling water is a general recipe for an infusion.

Nettle leaf supports the kidneys, helps prevent leg cramps, and contains vitamins A, C, D and K. It is also a source of calcium, phosphorus, iron and sulfur.

Dandelion leaf supports both the liver and the kidneys. It helps prevent preeclampsia and acts as a digestive aid. It is a source of vitamins A, B complex, C, and D.

Red raspberry leaf is a uterine toner, a digestive aid and a remedy for morning sickness.

Red clover leaves and blossoms are a source of calcium, magnesium and trace minerals. It supports the reproductive and endocrine system.

## Buying and Using Herbs

Certain herbs are contraindicated for use during pregnancy due to their harsh effect on certain organs. These include Goldenseal, Ephedra, Cotton root bark, Blue cohosh, Pennyroyal and Birthroot.

Buy dried herbs that have the strongest scent and color of their particular species. Faded herbs have not been properly stored and may not maintain their effectiveness, like any other medication.

An herbal tincture is a mixture of a fresh or dried herb in a liquid medium of alcohol or glycerin which extracts the effective portion of its chemicals. The mixture is strained and the resulting liquid stored for later use. Tinctures are administered by the dropperful. Knowledge of how the tincture was made aids proper usage. Those made from fresh, wild, or organically grown plants are best.

## Homeopathy in Pregnancy and Childbirth

Homeopathy is considered an "energy" medicine. Small, highly diluted doses of substances are given that, at full strength, are causes of the symptom being treated. Homeopathy treats the whole person by considering the personality and the factors that make the symptoms change. It sees significance in even minor symptoms. Homeopathic remedies work by stimulating self-healing rather than suppressing a symptom. Accurate advice should be obtained before attempting to use homeopathic remedies during pregnancy and childbirth.

Two common remedies are Arnica and Pulsatilla. Arnica Montana is used to treat bruising, shock, and trauma. It is used as a tablet or cream. It should not be applied to an open wound. Pulsatilla is used to treat hemorrhoids, varicose veins, and heartburn. It has also been used for apprehension and slow labor progress with ineffective contractions, emotional distress, and fainting.

## Motherwort Tincture, Skullcap Tincture, and Blessed Thistle Tonic

All of these herbs are said to keep the emotions calm during pregnancy.

Motherwort tincture calms without causing sleepiness. Five drops in a small glass of water helps the emotions balance about 15 minutes after ingestion. This can be taken as often as every 2 hours. However, it may become psychologically habit forming.

Skullcap tincture helps provide sleep. Up to 30 drops of a commercial tincture or 5 to 15 drops of fresh plant tincture 30 minutes before bed helps create a refreshing sleep. An infusion can help calm emotions. Two cups daily can be taken for several months.

Blessed Thistle tonic, along with Burdock and Sarsaparilla tonics, can be used occasionally as an emotion calming agent. This can be substituted for daily Raspberry Leaf infusion.

## Hydrotherapy

Hydrotherapy means, literally, water therapy. Water is used to deliver heat or cold to various areas of the body requiring analgesia or other treatment. In pregnancy, full immersion in a hot bath is not advisable due to possible danger to the fetus. Brief tepid baths are appropriate. Additionally, warm and cold compresses placed on affected body parts can increase circulation and analgesia. Hydrotherapy can increase the rate of healing and relaxation of aching muscles or bruising and sore tissues from birth.

## Shock

In childbirth, shock is most often caused by blood loss, which is also known as hypovolemic shock. Another possibility is septic shock. The symptoms of shock are:

- cool, clammy skin
- weak and rapid pulse
- dull eyes
- faintness
- weakness
- confusion

Occasionally, the mother will lose consciousness. Any delay in treating shock can result in multisystem organ failure and death. You must quickly determine the cause of the blood loss, make an effort to contain it, and stabilize the mother. In the meantime, the mother should be positioned flat on her back with her feet elevated. She should be kept warm without overheating, oxygen and fluids should be administered, and she should be encouraged to breathe deeply and calmly. Emergency medical services should be notified and the mother prepared for transport to a medical facility.

## Lidocaine

Lidocaine is a local anesthetic used when suturing a laceration. Lidocaine spray or gel is administered directly to the laceration then subcutaneous injections of 1% or 2% lidocaine are administered into the edges of the laceration.

- Wipe the top of the lidocaine bottle with alcohol
- Draw 5-10 cc's of air into the syringe and inject it into the bottle
- Draw 5-10 cc's of lidocaine into the syringe

Only 1 cc is administered in each location. The injections start at the top of the tear and descend. Do not insert the needle to the hilt. Slowly inject the medication, pulling back on the plunger at each injection site to ensure it has not entered a blood vessel. Wait for the anesthetic to take effect. It may not completely anesthetize the tissue; the mother will feel pressure and pulling but it should not be painful.

Lidocaine is also used for pudendal block.

## Ophthalmic Prophylaxis Ointment

Due to the prevalence of chlamydia and its asymptomatic nature, and the severity of gonorrheal infection, the risk to the newborn's eyes is such that prophylactic treatment with 0.5% erythromycin ointment, or other antibiotic, instilled into the eyes within a few hours of birth has been mandated by law in most states. Both pathogens may be transmitted to the newborn's eyes while passing through the birth canal. Gonorrhea can perforate the cornea and cause serious damage to the deeper eye structures. Chlamydia is a slightly milder infection but more common than gonorrheal infection. The mother may decline the prophylactic treatment in which case a waiver must be signed. The ointment is typically instilled from the inner to the outer canthus of each eye. Irrigation does not need to be performed afterwards. This prophylaxis should be delayed until after the first reactive period when the newborn must be able to see its parents.

## Rhogam

Rhogam is a plasma product given to RH negative mothers to prevent alloimmunization of their Rh positive newborn. Rhogam is specific for the D antibody, which a mother who is Rh negative will create whenever a fetal-maternal bleed has occurred. Since it is impossible to tell every such circumstance, Rhogam is given in every situation where the Rh negative mother has borne an Rh positive child; or if an Rh negative woman miscarries or has an abortion. Other procedures which may prompt the injection of Rhogam are chorionic villus sampling, amniocentesis, caesarian section, and any other procedure that could cause fetal-maternal transplacental hemorrhage (TPH). Rhogam suppresses the mother's production of antibodies in response to the Rh positive antigen from the baby. These antibodies can cause hemolytic disease of the newborn in subsequent pregnancies with an Rh positive fetus.

## Methergine, Pitocin, and Vitamin K

Methergine: an ergot derivative used to control uterine bleeding after delivery. It is offered as an oral medication or as an intramuscular injection and can be given when bleeding occurs or as a preventative. It promotes uterine contraction.

Pitocin (Oxytocin): similar to methergine and is given for the same condition. Pitocin causes uterine contractions which can help staunch or stop postpartum bleeding. Both methergine and pitocin are used when the placenta must be manually removed or when it properly separates but maternal bleeding does not cease.

Vitamin K: administered routinely to newborns to prevent hemorrhaging.

Vitamin K activates precursor proteins that in turn make blood clotting proteins. Injected Vitamin K stimulates clotting. It can also be found in alfalfa tablets which an expectant mother can take regularly in the last weeks of pregnancy to facilitate clotting after giving birth.

## Vitamin A, Vitamin C, Calcium, and Iron Risks

Vitamin A: is a teratogen in large doses which can cause birth defects. It can also affect the maternal liver.

Vitamin C: can cause increased absorption of iron which in turn causes problems when taken in excess.

Calcium: when taken in excessive quantities can affect kidney function and cause kidney stones as well as decrease absorption of iron, zinc and magnesium.

Iron: when taken in excessive quantities can also decrease absorption of zinc as well as copper and calcium.

It becomes evident that maintaining the appropriate levels of vitamins and minerals is a balancing act. If there is excess of one, another is usually impacted in some way, often to decrease absorption of that nutrient. It is prudent to take into consideration the diet, including any herbs or other supplements being ingested, before administering any additional vitamin or mineral supplementation.

## Nutritional Supplements

Prenatal Multivitamin: Contains appropriate levels of the vitamins most needed in pregnancy including increased folic acid and iron.

Vitamin C: Functions as a preventive antioxidant, often given to ward off infection.

Vitamin E: Functions as a non-specific chain breaking antioxidant. It is also occasionally used to relieve varicose veins.

Folic Acid: Prevents megaloblastic anemia in adults and neural tube defects in the fetus.

B-6: Functions as a coenzyme in the metabolism of amino acids and glycogen. It may also reduce morning sickness.

B-12: Reduces the occurrence of central nervous system damage in the newborn from a deficiency of B-12.

Iron: A component of hemoglobin which is used for oxygen transport in the red blood cell. Pregnancy creates an increased need for iron as well as other vitamins and minerals.

Calcium: Functions in blood clotting, muscle contraction, nerve transmission, and bone and tooth formation. It may also relieve pregnancy based hypertension.

Magnesium: Helps prevent preterm labor and stops preterm labor if it occurs.

## Ultrasounds

### *Risks*

Ultrasound imaging:

- Can give a false sense of wellness of the fetus
- Can give a false positive indications of abnormal conditions
- Ubiquitous use can cause an over-reliance on technology and an increase in health care costs

Randomized controlled studies have shown that, for a woman with no risk factors and a normal pregnancy, routine use of ultrasound made no difference in the outcome of the pregnancy as opposed to routine care and screening with manual methods by the health care practitioner. The quality of the information from the ultrasound can differ depending upon the expertise of the operator. A general ultrasonographer in a general radiology department may not as readily identify key components and anomalies as an ultrasonographer who routinely performs only pregnancy related scans and/or specializes in ultrasound for women with risks to their pregnancy. The National Institutes of Health have published a listing of indications for obstetrical ultrasound.

### *Benefits*

Ultrasound imaging:

- improves gestational age assessment with uncertain dates
- identifies fetal anomalies
- assesses fetal growth
- accurately identifies fetal demise, placental location, fetal position, and fetal number
- Amniotic fluid anomalies and pelvic masses are readily identified
- Gestational age assessment determines the course of ongoing management of prenatal care
- Identification of fetal anomalies by ultrasound can be done early enough in the pregnancy to allow the mother to terminate the pregnancy if she desires or to plan to care for a baby with abnormalities

- Conditions may be identified that can be corrected by intrauterine treatment or surgery
- Some studies of ultrasound show that alcohol and tobacco use decrease when ultrasound is performed

Ultrasound is best used in cases where the mother has risk factors that may decrease the chances of an optimal pregnancy outcome. The National Institute of Health has published a listing of indications for obstetrical ultrasound.

## Biophysical Profile

A BPP is indicated when IUGR, oligohydramnios, insulin-dependent diabetes, multiple pregnancy, pre-eclampsia, postdatism, non-reactive non-stress test, or a positive contraction stress test is known or suspected. Insulin dependent diabetics and post date pregnancies require a testing frequency of twice weekly while the other indications require once weekly. If there is a change in maternal status a BPP may need to be repeated. BPP is usually started at the earliest gestational age that the health care practitioner would consider delivery if the BPP showed an acidemic fetus. If oligohydramnios is noted cord compression is more likely to occur, therefore delivery is more likely to be recommended even though the rest of the BPP is within acceptable range. As the BPP score decreases the risk of complications increases. A score of 4/10 means that perinatal asphyxia has likely occurred and indicates a need for delivery. You must always consult with the physician whenever the scores are not reassuring.

### *Elements and Premise of the Biophysical Profile*

A biophysical profile (BPP) consists of a non-stress test using electronic fetal monitoring, and an ultrasound measurement of the volume of amniotic fluid and fetal activity. When a fetus is fully oxygenated and neurologically intact it has characteristics of muscle tone, gross movement and respiratory activity which are observable on ultrasound and the non-stress test will be reactive. Amniotic fluid volume is considered to be a measure of fetal renal function. If the fetus becomes hypoxic the characteristics mentioned above are negatively impacted. There is hypotonia, fetal breathing and movement is absent, and the non-stress test is non-reactive. There is a decreased blood flow to the fetal kidneys which reduces the volume of amniotic fluid. This presents as oligohydramnios in the uterus. Fetuses with anomalies, especially of the central nervous system, respiratory system or genitourinary system may have decreased BPP scores characteristic of their specific anomalies.

## Amni-Hook or Amnicot®

AROM or Artificial Rupture of the Membranes may be performed using this device, allowing labor to progress. To prevent cord prolapse, the baby's head should be low in the pelvic area, preferably zero (0) station or, in the event of a larger head, at -1 station. After putting on a sterile glove, sterile gel is placed on the fingers of the glove and the Amni-hook® or Amnicot® placed between the first two fingers with the tip protected. The mother is placed upright. At the end of a contraction, the gloved fingers are placed inside the vaginal canal and the hook pushed into the membranes. The handle is pressed down to lift the tip of the hook and the fingers drawn out slowly. Immediately afterwards heart tones should be checked and charted. This process should not be performed too early or complications due to prolonged rupture of the membranes may occur.

## Bag and Mask Resuscitator

Positive pressure ventilation using a resuscitation bag and mask is indicated when the newborn does not exhibit spontaneous, regular respirations or if the color is dusky after the newborn has been positioned on its back with the neck slightly extended and tactile stimulation has been ineffective. Flow-inflating bags use compressed oxygen to inflate and can deliver different pressures and concentrations of oxygen. This type should be adjusted to 5 cm $H_2O$ with a peak pressure of 30-40 cm $H_2O$ to avoid damage to newborn lungs. Self-inflating bags deliver a peak pressure of 30-40 cm $H_2O$ after which extra pressure is wasted to free air. They will not deliver high concentrations of oxygen unless a closed-ended reservoir is attached. This bag type should be used to deliver room air to a newborn if there is no source of compressed oxygen.

## Bulb Syringes, Hemostats, and Lancets

Bulb syringe: used to suction the neonate's nose and mouth on the perineum or immediately after birth. Completely expel the air from the bulb prior to insertion into the neonate's nose or mouth. Allow the bulb to expand then withdraw and empty it by forcing air out of the bulb again.

Hemostat: a scissor-like device with locking clamps used to control bleeding from a torn blood vessel by pinching the vessel closed without damaging the tissues. Use them in clamping the umbilical cord prior to cutting and in controlling bleeding while suturing lacerations.

Lancet: a sharp, pointed device used for punching a hole in the skin of the finger of an adult or the heel of a neonate to obtain blood for testing. Lancets can be either a flat, bladelike device with an arrow shaped tip or a needle-like tip mounted on a cylindrical plastic to be used manually or with a lancet device.

## Nitrazine Paper and DeLee® Device

Nitrazine paper: a blue-green paper test strip used for measuring pH. Impregnated with a specific dye, it is used to test the pH of vaginal secretions. Vaginal fluid is very acidic. If a neutral pH is found, amniotic fluid is present indicating ruptured membranes.

DeLee® (tube/mouth suction device): A DeLee device is a cup with a lid into which two small openings have been placed. Small pieces of tubing are attached, one to each opening. One piece of tubing is placed in the practitioner's mouth and the other piece of tubing is placed in the baby's mouth or nose. The practitioner applies gentle suction to her mouth tubing which then draws any matter from the baby's mouth or nose into the cup. This method of suctioning has fallen out of favor due to the small chance that infected blood or body fluid could reach the practitioner's mouth.

## Basic Suture Kit

The kit must contain:

- Two (2) needle holders. Five-inch Baumgartners are recommended. These have small, serrated tips that hold the needle without slipping. Hemostats should not be used as needle holders because of the difficulty in suturing well
- One (1) tissue forceps is needed, either Semkin-Taylor or Addsons, to hold and lift tissue; thumb forceps or dressing forceps are not suitable. The tissue forceps will not pinch or destroy membranes when used
- Two or three (2-3) mosquito hemostats should be included to control small bleeding vessels and never used for anything else
- One (1) pair of very sharp scissors to be used only for cutting suture material. These scissors should not be used during delivery or to cut the cord
- Four-by-four gauze pads or sponges
- Betadine solution
- suture material

All equipment should be kept sterile until the moment for use.

## Urinary Catheter

If the mother's bladder has become distended in second stage labor because she has been unable to empty it naturally, you may need to catheterize to empty it, preferably before the baby's head enters the true pelvis. Consider the following:

- whether the bladder is distended
- whether the mother has urinated in the past 2 hours
- whether the risk of a bladder infection is greater than the need to empty the bladder
- whether a complication is expected

A full bladder can cause discomfort or even become traumatized, especially if a labor complication ensues such as shoulder dystocia, which requires an empty bladder to manage. When the catheter is inserted at this point, the urethra is displaced by the fetal head and also conforms to the head's contours. The catheter must be guided in the direction of the urethra to avoid traumatizing the urethral wall.

## Vacutainer Type Blood Collection System

A vacutainer type blood collection system consists of a plastic sleeve with a narrow neck on one end to which a sterile, double-ended blood collection needle can be affixed. The end of the needle protruding from the holder is a beveled sterile needle for insertion into a patient's vein. The other end of the needle is contained inside the vacutainer with a flexible rubber diaphragm covering it. The needle is inserted into the vein and a collection tube is gently inserted into the sleeve and pushed onto the inner end of the needle. The tube will automatically fill to the appropriate level. Once full the tube is withdrawn and additional tubes can be filled. Any tube with anticoagulant or other additive should be mixed immediately upon withdrawal from the vacutainer. Most vacutainers are meant for one time use and come with an automatic needle cover for disposal in the appropriate container.

## Fetoscope and Dopplar

The fetoscope is a device used to monitor fetal heart tones and rate. The Allen fetoscope depends on bone conduction of the fetal heart sounds to the user's cranium. It produces muffled sounds of the fetal heart. It is difficult or impossible to hear the fetal heart with a fetoscope during a contraction. Close proximity to the mother's abdomen is required and positioning may cause problems with accuracy. The dopplar is now more commonly used due to increased accuracy and precision. It creates an electronic sound using ultrasound waves based on the movement of the fetal heart. The act of listening for the fetal heart tone in this manner is called auscultation. Intermittent auscultation is used not only to assess the heart rate but to note any variations beat-to-beat and to note any unexpected decelerations.

## Speculum

A speculum has two blades and a handle. It is inserted into the vagina and the two blades opened by use of a thumb-piece. Once opened, the intravaginal area and the cervix can be observed. There are several types of specula. The virginal speculum is the smallest and is meant for young girls and women with little coital experience. The Graves speculum, which has curved blades, comes in a standard size and a large size. The standard size is used for most women who are sexually active or who have borne at least one child. The large speculum is used for women with collapsing vaginal walls typically due to obesity or to grand multipara. The Pederson speculum is the same length as the Graves but the blades are narrower, flat, and best used for women who are sexually active but nulliparous or who have vaginas that are contracted by scarring, senescence, or radiation. Plastic specula are available.

## Laboratory Tests for All Pregnant Women

The menu of tests ordered for pregnant women can vary depending upon the policies of each facility. Some testing also varies with gestational age. You can be expected to collect blood and pap specimens during the first visit and exam. In general, the following tests are performed:

- Pap smear
- Gonococcal and Chlamydia samples (collected with the Pap smear)
- Blood Type and Rh factor with antibody screen/antibody titer
- Sickle cell screening
- Tuberculin test in high risk groups
- VDRL, RPR, or other syphilis serology test
- Hepatitis B surface antigen
- Rubella titer
- Varicella antibody screen
- Hemoglobin and hematocrit
- Urinalysis
- Diabetes screening (28 weeks)
- Group B Strep colonization (35-37 weeks)

All women should be offered HIV testing and alpha-feto protein or triple screen testing at 15 to 18 weeks.

## H&H, CBC and Blood Glucose Level

H&H (Hemoglobin/Hematocrit): a screening test for anemia. Hemoglobin should be 11 g/dl or greater and the hematocrit 33% or greater. Low values impact the oxygen carrying capacity of the mother's circulatory system.

Complete Blood Count (CBC): includes the hemoglobin and hematocrit. It also reports the number of red blood cells with their indices, the number of white blood cells with their type differential, and the number of platelets. A higher than normal white count may indicate the presence of an infection. Lower than normal platelet counts can result in bruising or extended bleeding.

Blood glucose level: also called blood sugar level, this test screens for diabetes. A normal fasting glucose level is less than 99 mg/dl. A higher reading indicates the possibility of gestational diabetes. A glucose tolerance test is then indicated. If gestational diabetes is diagnosed, closer monitoring of the mother's blood glucose is required.

## Blood Type and Rh Factors

An individual's blood type and Rh factor is inherited from the parents. There are four blood types: A, B, AB and O. Rh factor is an antigen that resides on the blood cell of Rh positive individuals. When the antigen is not present the individual is considered Rh negative. Knowledge of the maternal blood type and Rh factor is required for blood transfusion. Additionally, if the mother is Rh negative, there is a possibility of isoimmunization occurring which can cause the baby to become anemic due to hemolytic disease of the newborn. This rarely occurs in first births but subsequent fetuses are at risk of this disease if the mother is not treated with Rhogam within 72 hours of giving birth to an Rh positive baby. ABO incompatibility can also cause some jaundice in the baby if a type O mother receives type A or B blood cells from the fetus due to a fetal/maternal cross bleed.

## Single Dose Ampules and Multidose Vials

Single dose ampules of medication may be liquid or freeze dried. Reconstitute freeze dried medication with the accompanying liquid. Break the vial away from your face. If reconstitution is needed, draw up the required amount of liquid with a sterile syringe needle. After reconstitution use a new sterile needle to draw up the medication for injection. If the medication is already liquid, use a sterile needle and syringe to draw up the appropriate amount of medication and inject it into the patient.

Multidose vials may come liquid or dried. Use the same technique as above for reconstitution. Discard reconstituted medication vials after the expiry in certain number of hours. Multidose medication that comes as a liquid may be used until the expiry date as long as it is stored according to the manufacturer's instructions. Each time the multidose vial is used, wipe the diaphragm on the bottle with 70% alcohol. Use a sterile syringe needle each time the vial is entered.

## Pap Smear

A Pap smear is a diagnostic test in which cells from the cervix are obtained by gentle scraping and placed on a slide to be examined by a cytotechnologist. The test is a screen that describes and categorizes abnormal epithelial cells. On occasion other organisms are noted, such as *Candida*, *Trichomonas*, or cellular changes consistent with Herpes Simplex virus. None of these organisms is likely to need treatment and a Pap smear is not meant as a diagnostic tool for this use. If, however, it is noted that bacteria that are morphologically consistent with *Actinomyces spp*, a follow-up should be done if the woman has or had an IUD. *Actinomyces israelii* has been found to cause pelvic inflammatory disease. Pap smears should be performed early in pregnancy since hormonal changes may precipitate abnormal cell growth. A second smear should be taken 6 weeks post-partum to check for any differences from early pregnancy.

The Pap smear is the standard method of detecting cervical cancer. Cells from the endocervical region of the cervix are collected and processed. The slide is examined for abnormal signs. The report may include observations of various organisms such as Trichomonas or Candida and cellular changes due to inflammation or the presence of an IUD. Any abnormalities of the squamous and glandular cells and indications of carcinoma are reported. Any abnormal-appearing cervix, dysplasia, or cancer, ASC, repeated ASC, ACG, multiple unexplained inflammations, Pap smear reporting HPV infection history of intrauterine diethystilbesterol (DES) exposure should be referred for colposcopy. The gynecological culture is a method of diagnosing gonorrhea and Chlamydia. Gonorrheal infection during pregnancy has been linked to spontaneous abortion, very low birthweight, chorioamnionitis, postpartum endometritis, pelvic sepsis, and premature rupture of the membranes. Chlamydia in pregnancy has been linked to amnionitis and postpartum endometritis. Both infectious agents can infect the newborn as it transits the birth canal.

# Maternal Health Assessment

## Obstetrical History

A history of any obstetrical emergency such as placental abruption, fetal distress, postpartum hemorrhage, neonatal asphyxiation or shoulder dystocia and any transport to a hospital due to concerns during labor should be extensively documented and investigated. A history of childbirth losses also requires investigation as well as discussion of the mother's emotional attitude toward the loss. If a desire from a previous birth experience has not been met, the mother also may feel a sense of loss for that issue. If the mother has lost a child within two years of the current pregnancy, counseling and investigation of the physical and psychological impact should take place.

## Gynecological History

The following conditions may negatively impact the current pregnancy:

- A history of fibroids reduces the intrauterine space or disrupts placental implantation. Fibroids tend to increase greatly in size during pregnancy. They also increase the chance of postpartum hemorrhage. An ultrasound should be performed to learn the size and location of these benign uterine masses.
- Cone biopsies can cause scarring that reduces dilation.
- Cervical cauterization and cryosurgery may cause scarring.
- LEEP laser surgery may be implicated in cases of incompetent cervix and premature labor. Cervical changes may need to be monitored throughout the pregnancy and the mother educated about signs of premature labor.
- A contraceptive history of IUD use may cause anemia due to excess menstruation
- Pelvic inflammatory disease and IUD use can cause scarring of the uterine lining and result in ectopic pregnancy, irregular implantation of the placenta and third stage hemorrhage.
- The cervical os may be scarred.
- Oral contraceptive use can cause a folic acid deficiency.

## Other Types of Information

- Personal information is the beginning of the medical record, identifying an individual.
- Demographics can give clues to potential age or ethnically related complication.
- Information regarding religion can identify cultural or religious needs.
- The mother's occupation determines when she stops working. If she is in a physically demanding job she will likely need to stop earlier than if she has a desk job. Her occupation may increase her environmental exposure to toxins.
- Marital and economic status can reveal stressors if the mother is single, estranged, or financially insecure.
- Educational level determines what level to communicate on. A lack of education may lead to misunderstandings and inadvertent non-compliance.
- Any changes in health or behavior can be cause for concern if it is a degradation of health or abnormal behavior. A woman's evaluation of her own health and nutrition are valuable markers of commitment to the pregnancy and of her awareness of her health and diet.

## Family and Psychosocial History

A complete family history can indicate a predisposition toward conditions that may impact the pregnancy such as a tendency towards diabetes, hypertension, anemia, or other conditions requiring the attention of a specialist. Genetic issues may also be revealed such as the tendency for thalassemia, a condition more often seen in a particular ethnic group.

An effective psychosocial history may be difficult to obtain, particularly as psychological issues are uncomfortable to confront. There are many different ways that pregnancy and motherhood can impact an individual. Some of these ways are revealed when the reasons for a home birth are discussed. The mother may be affected by:

- Previous pregnancies, abortions, miscarriages, abusive relationships or the existence of previous children
- Societal expectations of motherhood that seem unattainable or unwanted
- Unreasonable expectations of herself.

Any psychological stress can create an issue with the pregnancy and birth if not addressed and resolved early.

### Menstrual and Sexual History

The menstrual history includes the cycle length and the normal volume of menstrual flow. A cycle length that is longer or shorter than the average of 28 days can impact the estimated due date. If the mother states that her periods are normally heavier than the last menstrual period before pregnancy it could mean the conception took place as much as a month earlier than originally believed and the LMP was implantation bleeding. Risky sexual behavior exposes the mother to sexually transmitted diseases and if the behavior is still taking place it exposes an issue with the mother's commitment to the pregnancy and birth. Counseling and education may help the mother change this behavior. This is also true of other personally risky behaviors such as smoking or taking illegal drugs and sharing needles, thereby risking exposure to blood borne diseases.

### Physical Exam

The physical exam can be a way of gaining trust with the new client and to check for underlying conditions that may impact pregnancy. A physical exam typically includes a "review of systems" (ROS) which is a structured investigation of past or current symptoms or complaints. ROS during the physical exam eliminates repetition but can cause information to become disconnected. Immediately prior to the exam thoroughly wash and warm your hands. Keep nails trimmed to avoid scratching the client. Touch to the client gently but firmly to avoid tickling and communicate respect for the client's body. Explain each touch first. Minimize the need for movement by the client. The exam should proceed the same way for every client to avoid missing anything and should proceed from head to toe. Communicate all findings to the client whether normal, abnormal or in need of confirmation by another examiner such as a physician.

The following elements comprise a thorough physical exam:

- general appearance and condition of skin
- baseline weight and height
- vital signs
- examine (HEENT) including the hair and scalp
- examine lymph glands of the upper body
- assess the breasts and the mother's knowledge of and compliance with self-breast examination techniques
- examine the torso and extremities for abrasions, bruising, unusual growths, or moles
- baseline reflexes

- auscultate heart and lungs
- palpate the abdomen noting any scarring
- internal pelvic landmarks and measurements
- assess Pap smear and gynecological culture results
- bimanually determine uterine and ovarian size
- assess vulva, vagina, cervix, perineum, and anus
- assess kidney pain or CVAT results
- assess joint pain, muscular strength, spinal straightness, symmetry, and posture
- assess the vascular system including indications of edema, varicosities or thrombophlebitis

## Vital Signs

Take vital signs at every visit, including baseline readings at the first physical exam. Vital signs include temperature, pulse, respirations, and blood pressure. Height is taken at the first physical exam but is rarely checked again. Assume the woman is in a relaxed state and has not exerted herself in the past few minutes. Increased temperature indicates infection although it may also be a symptom of dehydration. The source of any infection should be investigated. Increased pulse rate may be due to anxiety or exertion, or it may be a sign of infection, dehydration or shock. An increased respiratory rate can also be due to anxiety, shock or infection. If accompanied by coughing or wheezing, asthma or respiratory infection may be to blame. Increased or decreased blood pressure can indicate a hypertensive disorder of pregnancy or shock, in that order.

## Observations of Skin and Hair During Physical Exam

ROS includes an exam of the skin for pruritus, rashes, moles, lesions, tendency towards bruising, hirsutism and the type of skin: oily or dry. It includes and exam of the hair for hair loss, reasons for wearing a wig, whether there is a scalp infection, dandruff or lice, and the type: oily or dry.

Document and investigate abnormal temperature, color (pallor, cyanosis, pigmentation, and jaundice), moles, scars, turgor, rashes, lesions, bruises, tumors, and patterns of injury on the skin. Examine the hair and scalp for bald spots, lumps, hair pattern, and infections. The skin and hair can indicate variety of conditions:

- hypothyroidism causes dry skin and hair
- a pattern of injury may indicate domestic violence, abuse, a balance problem, or self-mutilation
- changes in moles over time in the size, shape, or color of the mole can indicate melanoma
- cyanosis indicates a respiratory or cardiac problem
- jaundice may indicate a liver condition

## ROS and Examination of the Head

ROS for the head includes determination of the incidence of headaches:

- location, duration, time of day of occurrence
- type of pain, frequency
- any known causes, any medications or other remedies taken and the effectiveness
- other symptoms associated with them

ROS also includes dizziness, syncope, and sinusitis. Other observations include:

- the size, shape, contour and symmetry of the head
- the facial symmetry

- the location of the facial structures
- facial tenderness over the sinuses
- involuntary movements

Syncope can be vasovagal, cardiogenic (often from arrhythmias), orthostatic, and neurogenic. It may also be due to certain medications. The most common types of headaches are migraines and tension headaches. Sinusitis is often caused by a bacterial infection in the sinus due to sinus blockage and subsequent inability to drain. Common bacterial causes are *Staphylococcus sp.*, especially *S. aureus*, and *Hemophilus influenzae.*

## ROS for the Eyes

ROS for the eyes should include a discussion of any blurring of vision, scotomata, diplopia, spots before the eyes, flashing lights, pressure or pain, injuries, diseases or conditions, photophobia, discharge, redness, burning, lacrimation, the presence of corrective lenses, and the patient's own evaluation of her visual health. Other observations include whether the eyelids are abnormally closed, edematous, have signs of infection, masses, lesions, ptosis, matting in or absence of eyelashes, involuntary eye movements, observation of the lacrimal ducts for infection or tenderness, the color of the sclera and lower conjunctival sac, any abrasions or opacities of the lens or cornea, strabismus, parallel movement, papillary reaction to light, protrusion of the eyeball, the size, shape and equal appearance of the eyes. It also includes an ophthalmoscope exam for red reflex, optic disc, any hemorrhage, papilledema, retinal vessels, macula and fovea.

## Scotomata, Diplopia, Photophobia, Lacrimation, and Strabismus

Scotomata: an island like blind spot in the visual field. There are many different types of scotomata: annular, absolute, arcuate, central, centrocecal, color, eclipse, flittering, negative, peripheral, physiological, positive, relative, ring, and scintillating.

Diplopia: double vision, or, more formally, two images of an object seen at the same time. There are several types of diplopia: binocular, crossed, homonymous, monocular, uncrossed, and vertical.

Photophobia: also called photodysphoria, this is an intolerance, or sensitivity, to light.

Lacrimation: the secretion of tears. It may become excessive.

Strabismus: an optical disorder where the optic axes cannot be directed to the same object. It is commonly called crossed eyes. There are several types: unilateral, alternating, constant, and periodic.

## Thyroid

The thyroid is part of ROS of the neck. Abnormal symptoms include: enlargement, excessive sweating, dry skin or hair, fatigue or excessive energy. Common laboratory tests for diagnosis of thyroid disease are TSH, Free T4 and Serum T3. Total T4 is not as significant.

Hyperthyroidism means TSH is low or absent and T3 and Free T4 are increased. Grave's Disease, an autoimmune disease, is the most common type. The thyroid is enlarged and tender with optical symptoms. Another less common cause of hyperthyroidism is high hCG in hydatidiform moles. Treatment alterations during pregnancy keep Free T4 levels in the high-normal range.

In hypothyroidism TSH is elevated, most commonly due to Hashimoto's thyroiditis, an autoimmune disease. Postpartum thyroiditis presents as hyperthyroidism first, then hypothyroidism. Recovery is spontaneous but may recur in future pregnancies and may increase the risk of thyroid disease in the future. L-Thyroxine is the typical medical treatment.

## ROS for the Mouth

ROS for the mouth includes toothaches, bleeding, lesions, pain, or edema of the gums, lips, mouth, or tongue, extractions and dentures, and difficulty with swallowing or chewing. Other observations include breath odor, color and symmetry of lips and tongue, whether the palate is intact, the color of the mucus membrane and gum, and any signs of infection. Dental work should be completed prior to conception, especially if it involves radiation exposure, sedation, gum surgery, or anesthesia. Significant periodontal disease can cause premature labor and birth. If gums are manipulated during pregnancy, bleeding is increased due to the increased vascularity caused by the pregnancy. Between pregnancy and any time spent breastfeeding, there may be significant delay in dental care if it is not performed prior to conception.

## Mucus Membranes

The mucus membranes are found in the nose, mouth, eyes, and other internal areas that can be exposed to the environment. Mucus formed within the membranes and nonpathogenic organisms form another level of resistance to infection of the body. Examination of the mucus membranes should note:

- degree of moisture
- hyperemia
- pallor
- cyanosis
- pigmentation
- lesions
- hemorrhage

Anemias will cause pallor; temporary pallor can be caused by shock, vasomotor spasm, or severe hemorrhage. Pallor occurring in alternation with flushing indicates aortic regurgitation. Hyperemia, or excessive redness, is caused by different pathologies depending on the tissue. Redness in the mouth can be due to tooth decay, stomatitis or trauma. Redness in the nose can be caused by ulceration, inflammation, or rhinitis. Dry membranes indicate fever, chronic gastritis, liver disturbances, shock, prostration, fatigue, dehydration, and use of certain drugs.

## Lymph Glands

Lymph glands in the neck, chest and under the arms are checked for swelling. This is often done as part of the breast exam. The supraclavicular and infraclavicular regions are palpated for the subclavian nodes. The anterior axilla area is palpated for the pectoral nodes while the posterior axilla area is palpated for the subscapular nodes. The middle of the axilla area contains the central axillary nodes and the upper arm has the lateral brachial nodes. Any palpable node is cause for concern and should be referred to a physician for investigation. Occasionally infections distal to nodes can cause enlargements of those nodes. If palpable nodes are found in the axilla area, the fingers and hand of that side should be examined for abrasions and cuts around the cuticles and fingernails. Consultation with a physician to confirm this diagnosis is required.

### Normal Variations in Breast Tissue

Breast masses are more difficult to diagnose due to the changes in the breast during pregnancy. Normal variations in a pregnant woman include:

- increase in size, possible tingling, tenderness
- increased general coarse nodularity and lobularity
- colostrum discharge as early as 6 weeks gestation
- Montgomery's follicles
- enlargement and increased erection of the nipples
- broadening and increased pigmentation of the areola
- dilated subcutaneous veins
- vascular spiders on upper chest
- striae of the breasts

A supportive, well-fitted bra, gently cleaning dried colostrum from nipples, and assist everting flat or inverted nipples give comfort in pregnancy and postnatal breastfeeding. Colostrum expression is another presumptive sign of pregnancy. It also helps prove to an anxious mother that there is something to feed the newborn in her breasts if she is uncertain.

### Breast Exam by Health Care Practitioner

Observe the breasts with arms by sides, arms raised overhead, and with hands pressed against hips or palms pressed together under the chin. Observe the breasts while the client is bent forward from the hips with arms extended toward the examiner.

Next palpate the supraclavicular and infraclavicular regions for the subclavian nodes; palpate the axilla; inspect the nipple epithelium. Lastly, palpate the breasts on a supine client.

Refer all abnormal findings to a physician:

- asymmetry in breast contour
- retraction signs
- nipple deviation or retraction
- shrunken breast
- edema
- dilated subcutaneous veins
- redness or heat in non-postpartal breasts
- ulcerations
- excessive breast elevation and asymmetry with contracted pectoral muscles
- palpable nodes
- erosion
- ulceration
- thickening
- roughness, redness, or crusting of the nipples (in a non-breastfeeding woman)
- coarse, granular nodularity in a localized area
- loss of elasticity of the tissue or nipple with increased firmness or thickening of skin
- any mass

## Self Breast Examination Technique

Examine the breasts in a mirror, first with arms down then with them up, to determine the normal look of the breasts and to check for:

- dimpling, puckering, or bulging of the skin
- an inverted nipple or a nipple that has changed position
- redness, soreness, rash or swelling

While at the mirror, squeeze each nipple gently to check for discharge of any color. Check the feel of the breasts first while supine then while upright, using the left hand to check the right breast and vice versa. Raise the opposing arm above the head. Examine the breast with the fingers together and flat, using a firm touch. Examine the entire breast including the nipple from collarbone to abdomen and cleavage to armpit using a pattern that covers the entire area. Palpate all tissue, from just under the skin down to the ribcage. The upright exam may more easily be performed in the shower on wet or soapy skin.

## ROS of the Cardiorespiratory System

ROS for the cardiorespiratory system includes dyspnea, orthopnea, tachypnea, wheezing, cough, pleurisy, sputum production, cyanosis, dependent edema, night sweats, palpitations, hemoptysis, chest pain, stridor, history of respiratory infections, contact with tuberculosis, results and date of latest chest x-ray, known abnormalities of the heart rate or rhythm, history of rheumatic heart disease, anemia, hypertension, and coronary artery disease (CAD).

Dyspnea is a lack of air resulting in labored or difficult breathing. Breathing may be audible with retracted intercostal spaces, and cyanosis. Orthopnea is labored breathing while supine. Tachypnea is abnormally rapid respiration.

Pleurisy is the inflammation of the pleura and can be primary or secondary; unilateral, bilateral or local; acute or chronic, fibrinous, serofibrinous, or purulent.

Hemoptysis is the expulsion or expectoration of blood from the larynx, trachea, bronchi or lungs. Small amounts may occur in several illnesses that may irritate these areas. Stridor is a high-pitched sound occurring on inspirations indicating an upper airway obstruction.

## Scars/Bruises, Linea Nigra, and Abdominal Striae

Examine the abdomen for scars and bruises to obtain information regarding the woman's health and potential problems. Scars and bruises on the abdomen should be satisfactorily explained by the mother. They may be evidence of physical abuse. In the case of scars, a caesarian scar is particularly important to note to determine if the mother is wishing to VBAC. Note any appendectomy scar so that any right side pain will not be misdiagnosed. The linea nigra and the abdominal striae are *presumptive* physical signs of pregnancy.

## CVAT

CVAT can be an indication of pyelonephritis, which is an inflammation of the kidney and renal pelvis, most typically due to a urinary tract infection traveling up from the bladder. The most common bacterial infection is due to *E. coli*. Treatment for pyelonephritis includes IV antibiotics. If successfully treated, there is no adverse effect to the pregnancy.

Palpation for CVAT should be performed when assessing first trimester bleeding. The costovertebral angle is formed at the junction of the twelfth rib and the paravertebral muscles. Any pain in this area is typical of renal disease. CVAT is elicited during exam by lightly striking the woman's back, using the ulnar surface of the fist, from the midportion of the scapular area to the midportion of the buttock area. Ensure the CVA is struck on the way. Any report of pain during this exam should be investigated.

## Deep Tendon Reflexes

Tapping a tendon briskly can cause a brief muscle stretch. Baseline reflexes are needed to compare for changes in future reflex exams. If the reflexes are hyperactive, there may be a disease of the upper motor neuron or pyramidal tract. Some diseases can cause hypoactive reflexes. Reflexes are evaluated according to a scale from zero to 4+ with zero meaning the reflex was absent and 4+ indicating hyperactivity. Reflexes at either extreme, zero or 4+ are abnormal and the patient should be referred to a physician. Reflexes should be symmetrical from one side to the other. Clonus is rapid, repetitive, rhythmical, involuntary contraction and relaxation of a muscle when it is sharply stretched and the stretch is maintained in either flexion or extension. It is only present when there is central nervous system disease. It is typical of upper motor neuron disease. Check for clonus If hyperreflexia is found.

## Brachioradialis, Quadriceps, and Gastrocnemius-Soleus Deep Tendon Reflexes

Brachioradialis reflex: The radius is used to elicit this response rather than a tendon directly. The patient's arm is slightly flexed, the hand slightly bent at the wrist, and the arm rested on lap or abdomen. The elbow and forearm should flex.

Quadriceps (knee-jerk) reflex: The patellar tendon below the patella is struck. The leg is flexed. The knee should extend and the leg should jerk.

Gastrocnemius-soleus (ankle-jerk) reflex: The Achilles' tendon above the heel is struck. The leg is flexed at the knee and the foot is dorsiflexed. Plantar flexion of the foot at the ankle should be observed.

## Biceps and Triceps Deep Tendon Reflexes

Biceps reflex: The tendon of the biceps brachii in the bend of the elbow is struck. The patient's arm is flexed and rested on her lap or the examiner's arm. The elbow, arm and forearm should flex; the hand should supinate.

Triceps reflex: The tendon of the triceps brachii on the back of the upper arm above the elbow is struck. The patient's arm is flexed and the elbow held in the patient's opposing hand. The elbow and forearm should extend and the arm should adduct.

## Pelvimetry

Pelvimetry is the practice of manually measuring internal structures of the pelvis during a pelvic exam to assess possible issues with birthing. All measurements are in centimeters.

First, the depth of the sacral curve is measured. It is found by locating the coccyx and tracing the sacral curve up toward the sacral promontory. Here the size of the pelvic inlet is assessed. Upon reaching the sacral promontory the diagonal conjugate is measured. From this measurement is extracted the obstetric conjugate, the inlet dimension the fetus must move through. A measurement of 10.5 cm or greater is adequate. The contour of, and distance between, the ischial spines is measured next. The amount of sharpness and protrusion is noted then the distance between the spines, called the interspinous diameter, is measured. 10.5 cm is adequate. The angle or width of the pubic arch is assessed next followed by the outlet dimension, or intertuberous diameter. An adequate measurement is 8.5 cm or greater.

## Female Pelvic Bones and Ligaments

There are three pelvic bones: the innominate (hip) bones (2), the sacrum (1) and the coccyx (1). The innominate bones are composed of the ilium, the ischium, and the pubic bone. The ischium contains an inward projection called the ischial spine. The station of the fetal head is estimated in relation to this spine during labor.

There are four pelvic joints: the symphysis pubis (1), the sacroiliac joints (2) and the sacrococcygeal joint (1). During pregnancy, the ligaments soften due to estrogenic activity and move to make room for the fetal head during birth. The symphysis pubis may separate before birth, causing discomfort while walking. The pelvic joints are held together by the interpubic ligaments at the symphysis pubis, the sacroiliac ligaments and the sacrococcygeal ligaments. Two other important ligaments are the sacrotuberous ligament and the sacrospinous ligament which cross the sciatic notch and form the posterior wall of the pelvic outlet.

## Pelvic Inclination

The pelvis is on an incline when the female is standing erect. The line between the sacral promontory and the top of the symphysis pubis forms a 60 degree angle with the floor. A line from the center of the sacrum and the center of the symphysis pubis forms a 30 degree angle with the floor. At the outlet, the angle of inclination is 15 degrees. In a recumbent position, these angles would be formed with a vertical surface rather than the floor; you should be cognizant of this when performing an abdominal examination. The curve of Carus is formed when a curved line is imagined exactly half-way between the anterior pelvic wall and the posterior pelvic canal. Familiarity is required of this structure when examining the vagina and when assisting in birth.

## True Pelvis

The true pelvis is the bony opening through which the fetus passes during birth. It is formed by a brim, a cavity and an outlet.

Fixed points on the pelvic brim are landmarks. Beginning from the posterior the landmarks are as follows:

- sacral promontory
- sacral ala or wing
- sacroiliac joint
- iliopectineal line
- iliopectineal eminence
- superior ramus of the pubic bone
- upper inner border of the body of the pubic bone
- the upper inner border of the symphysis pubis

Three diameters of the brim are measured. One, the obstetrical conjugate, is about 11 cm from the sacral promontory to the posterior border of the upper surface of the symphysis pubis. This is the space through which the fetal head must pass.

The obstetrical outlet portion of the pelvic outlet is formed by the narrow pelvic strait and the anatomical outlet. The anteroposterior diameter, a line from the lower border of the symphysis pubis to the sacrococcygeal joint measuring 13 cm, indicates the available space during delivery.

## Four Pelvic Types

Gynecoid: Considered "ideal" for bearing children. The brim is rounded and the forepelvis is roomy. The ischial spines are blunt, sciatic notch rounded, and sub-pubic angle 90 degrees. The woman's build and height is average. Smaller women may have a justo minor pelvis, exactly the same as gynecoid but with smaller measurements.

Android: Least suited to childbearing. The brim is heart-shaped; the forepelvis is narrow. The ischial spines are prominent and sub-pubic angle less than 90 degrees. The woman's build and height is short and heavy.

Anthropoid: Typically no issues for delivery. The brim is long and oval, with the anteroposterior diameter longer than the transverse. The ischial spines are not prominent, a very wide sciatic notch and sub-pubic angle. The woman's build is tall with narrow shoulders.

Platypelloid: Typically no issues for delivery. The brim is kidney shaped; the pelvis flat. The anteroposterior diameter is decreased; the transverse increased. The ischial spines are blunt with a wide sub-pubic angle and sciatic notch.

## Female Reproductive System with and Without Pregnancy

The pituitary releases GnRH and the anterior pituitary releases FSH and LH. FSH influences follicles within the ovaries to enlarge and estrogen levels increase. LH is produced a few days after FSH' when both levels peak, the follicle ruptures and ovulation occurs. Estrogen levels increase causing FSH production to stop. Progesterone levels rise and cause FSH and LH levels to fall. If the released ovum is not fertilized, it degenerates in 14 days and the cycle begins again.

The ovum moves along the Fallopian tubes. It can be fertilized by only a single sperm. The gametes merge to convert the ovum into a zygote. Once the zygote reaches the uterus in the form of a blastocyst, the outer layer becomes the placenta and chorion, and the inner portion becomes the fetus, amnion and umbilical cord. The blastocyst adheres to the uterine wall and is embedded into the endometrium (implantation). The zygote becomes an embryo until 8 weeks post conception when it becomes a fetus.

## Cervical Exam

Chadwick's sign in pregnancy is indicated by a bluish color of the cervix caused by increased vascularity. A non-pregnant cervix is pink. Growths, lesions, nodules, ulcerations, masses, polyps, erosions, and infected nabothian cysts are abnormal. Refer to physician. Cervicitis, an inflammation of the cervix, is typically caused by an irritation, injury, or infection. Cervicitis presents with hypertrophy, edema, discharge, and friability. Deviation of the uterus to one side can indicate pelvic masses or uterine adhesions. Eversion is caused by pressure on the vaginal fornices by the speculum and it should disappear if the speculum is moved back. Ectopy occurs in multiparous women or women using oral contraceptives. The size and shape of the os are impacted by childbirth. If lacerations of the os are extensive the cervix may be incompetent. Parity affects the patulousness of the cervix. The nulligravid cervix is closed. A multiparous cervix is open to a larger degree with each birth. Dilation can also be observed at this time.

## Uterus and Ovaries During a Pelvic Exam

The uterus is palpated bimanually. One hand is placed on the abdomen between the umbilicus and the symphysis pubis. Two vaginal fingers should be placed to either side of the cervix, pressed on top of it and the cervix pushed downwards with the backs of the fingers. The tips of the fingers are pushed upwards to feel the shape, size and contour of the uterus. A multiparous uterus is larger than a nulliparous uterus. An enlarged uterus can indicate pregnancy or tumors. Normal nulliparous size is 5.5 to 8 cm long, 3.5 cm wide, and 2 to 2.5 cm thick. A multiparous uterus is slightly larger. The ovaries are also palpated at this time. Normal ovaries during childbearing years are 2.5 to 5 cm long, 1.5 to 3 cm wide, and 0.5 to 1.5 cm thick. After menopause ovarian size decreases significantly.

### Uterine Abnormalities

The uterus can be malformed due to the failure of the Müllerian ducts to fuse correctly. This can result in several abnormalities: a double uterus with a double vagina, a double uterus with a single vagina, a bicornate uterus, and other deformities depending on where the fusion fails. The difficulty in pregnancy depends on the severity of the abnormality. If the uterus can still stretch to accommodate a full size fetus, the pregnancy may not be endangered. If it cannot, premature labor, abnormal lie of the fetus, and abortion may result. In the case of a double uterus, the fetus takes up one horn while the other remains empty. The empty horn enlarges under hormonal influence and can obstruct the birth canal. In this case, a caesarian section will be required.

### External Genitalia, Vagina, Cervix, Perineum, and Anus

The external genitalia, or vulva, are examined prior to the pelvic and speculum exams. The mons is observed for hair growth pattern and pediculosus. The labia majora and perineum are checked for swelling, edema, cysts, inflammation, dermatitis, irritation, discoloration, tenderness, lesions, vesicles, ulcerations, crusting, or condylomata. Investigate and refer to a physician. Varicosities and episiotomy or perineal laceration scars should be considered when creating the birth plan. The labia minora is checked for inflammation, irritation, discoloration, herpetic vesicles, chancre, fistulas or fissures which must be referred to a physician. The clitoris is checked for adhesions and enlargement; the urethral orifice is checked for irritation or dilation (possible repeated UTIs or insertion of foreign objects), and for growths or fistulas, all to be referred to a physician. The vaginal introitus is also inspected for all of the above problems and physician consultations sought for abnormal growths, fistulas, fissures, and uterine prolapse.

# Prenatal

## Maternal Psychological Changes

### *First Trimester*

The emotions and psychological balance of a pregnant woman are very changeable. She can be very sensitive, introspective, vulnerable and dependent. The first trimester is known as the "period of adjustment"; the mother must accept that she is pregnant. Most will be disappointed, anxious, depressed and/or unhappy about the pregnancy, no matter how prepared they were to become pregnant. You must discuss these feelings and their ubiquitousness. These feelings often persist until the pregnancy is accepted. Most mothers want to wait until this trimester ends to notify others of the pregnancy. Many mothers also begin to think about weight gain at this time, either as a happy confirmation of pregnancy or another element to hide from others. The mother often wants repeated evidence of the pregnancy. Divulge the pelvic findings; it will be appreciated. She, and her partner if possible, should be counseled that her libido may decrease during this time.

### *Second Trimester*

During the second trimester, or "the period of radiant health", the mother feels good but is at her most introspective. This trimester is divided in to prequickening and postquickening. Quickening makes the pregnant woman the most aware she has been of her impending motherhood. Her primary adjustment is to discover her own mothering identity. Prior to quickening, she will re-examine her relationship with her own mother and divine those qualities she will keep or reject. After quickening, the social circle of the mother changes to include more new mothers or others who are pregnant. Relationships change. Some grief is felt. The baby is now seen as a separate entity and the woman begins to focus on the baby instead of herself. In addition, her libido may increase as may her ability to feel sexual satisfaction.

### *Third Trimester*

The third trimester is the "time of watchful waiting". The mother becomes anxious both for the baby's arrival and worried about premature labor. Visible preparation begins, including choosing names, preparing the baby's room, and receiving gifts. Now is the time of fear about death and abnormalities, and pain during childbirth. The mother may worry that she won't recognize labor or that the baby is unable to come through the birth canal. The mother may grieve the loss of attention as well as the closeness of the baby once it is born. There is also physical discomfort affecting her emotions, feeling fat or awkward. The mother's partner should be made aware that loving, non-sexual contact is needed to emotionally support her.

## Infection

Infections are caused by pathogenic microorganisms such as bacteria, viruses, fungi, parasites, protozoans, and rickettsia. Infection during pregnancy can directly impact the mother and directly and indirectly impact the fetus. Systemic infections can cause chills, sweats, fever, malaise, and sometimes headache, muscle or joint pain, or changes in mental status. Localized infections can cause tissue swelling and redness, tenderness, heat, and loss of function. The fetus is indirectly impacted when the mother is too ill to take in proper nutrition or maintain proper hydration. The fetus can be directly impacted by certain infections that cause congenital abnormalities.

Infections must be differentially diagnosed to determine appropriate treatment. Due to increasing numbers of drug resistant bacteria any bacterial pathogen may require additional study to determine an effective antibiotic. Prescribing antibiotics for a viral infection is ineffective, may be detrimental to the patient, and may increase antibiotic resistance of bacteria that are also present.

### Blood Pressure Norms

Maternal blood pressure should be checked and charted at each visit. The systolic reading (first number) indicates the pressure in the arteries when the heart is actively pumping and indicates the cardiovascular tolerance for exertion. The diastolic reading (second number) is the pressure when the heart is at rest and indicates baseline intravascular tension. Normal blood pressure during pregnancy is in the range of 90/50 to 140/90. In pregnancy, blood pressure may be somewhat elevated due to tension or excitement. However, blood pressure higher than 130/80 may indicate undiagnosed essential hypertension. A steady increase from the baseline may indicate the need for stress reduction techniques. If edema or proteinuria accompanies the increase in blood pressure, preeclampsia may be indicated requiring immediate referral to the consulting physician.

### Appropriate Weight Gain

During the first visit, the mother's weight should be checked and charted along with her pre-pregnancy weight and a note of the total gain to date. If the mother's pre-pregnancy weight was appropriate for her frame and height, she should gain an average of one pound a week. It should be emphasized to her that an ample weight gain is required for fetal health and maternal endurance during pregnancy and labor. However, the weight gain should not be overdone as gaining too much weight can also cause complications, not only during pregnancy and childbirth but afterwards since the gained weight may be hard to lose. Generally, the following weight gain is accepted as appropriate:

- Underweight women should gain 27 to 40 pounds
- Normal weight women should gain 25 to 35 pounds
- Overweight women should gain 15 to 25 pounds
- Obese women should gain less than 15 pounds

### Weight Gain Issues for Pregnant Women

Underweight women may gain more weight during pregnancy while overweight women should gain less. By 20 weeks approximately 10 pounds should be gained with one pound a week after that. If more weight is gained than expected and it is not due to a growth spurt of the fetus, the mother may have changed her dietary habits due to unsound nutritional information. Sometimes there is a perceived need to watch weight because of a partner's attitude or simply physical discomfort with extra food intake. Nutritional information, patient urging to eat healthy foods for the baby's sake, and working with the mother to find alternatives to favorite but unhealthy foods may put her back on track. An outline of poor consequences if this plan is not followed may increase cooperation. Pregnancy may cause eating disorders to recur and a history of eating disorders may require the services of a specialist.

### Bowel or Urination Habits

In the first trimester, the weight and shape of the uterus changes to increase pressure on the bladder, causing the feeling of urgency to urinate. In the third trimester, because the engaging part of the fetus has descended and the enlarged uterus crowds the other organs, the bladder loses the room to expand and the need to urinate more frequently occurs. In addition, when edema occurs, the fluid drains during the night and increases the need to urinate during the night, interrupting sleep. Education is the only remedy to this issue, teaching causes and suggesting limiting fluids directly before bedtime.

Constipation may develop during pregnancy. Peristalsis is slowed during the third trimester by progesterone. The increasing size of the uterus may also compress the bowel and limit peristaltic movement. Adequate fluids, rest and fiber, and mild laxative foods such as prunes and warm liquids, with the addition of gentle exercise can keep the bowel moving and regular.

### Changes in Sleep Patterns

Pregnancy increases the demands on the body and adequate rest is required whenever possible to maintain the health and energy of the mother. Women who may never have napped prior to pregnancy may now find themselves in need of at least one nap during the day of about 30 to 60 minutes. As the pregnancy progresses, it may become more difficult to obtain uninterrupted sleep due to the need to urinate during the night due to bladder constriction and edematous fluid drain and other discomforts. The distension and weight of the uterus, the activity of the fetus, muscular aches due to the pregnancy may all combine to disrupt or inhibit sleep. Remedies include warm baths, a warm drink such as milk prior to bed, and techniques of relaxation may all help, if not ensure a good night's sleep, at least make getting more sleep easier.

### Serum Glucose, Hemoglobin and Hematocrit

The total blood volume in a singleton pregnancy can increase between 30% and 50% with increases above 50% in multiple gestation. The majority of the volume increase is an increase in the plasma volume which causes a hemodilution effect. This in turn causes the hematocrit to decrease as the ratio of red blood cells to plasma changes. The most significant decrease in hematocrit occurs between weeks 24 and 32. After 32 weeks the hemodilution effect stabilizes. Unless the mother is diabetic in any form, the normal serum glucose levels of a pregnant woman will not differ from a non-pregnant one. Gestational diabetes will cause the serum glucose to remain elevated longer than normal and may cause the levels to become more elevated than normal when ingesting a standard load of glucose.

### Breast Condition in Breastfeeding

The breast size does not indicate ability to produce sufficient breastmilk. Gigantomastia and micromastia may indicate underlying issues and can contraindicate the ability to breastfeed. Trauma to the chest and/or breast may affect nipple patency or the ability to produce breastmilk. Biopsy, surgery, or injury to the breast may impact the nerve tissue and/or the ducts and decrease the ability to breastfeed.

Classification of inverted nipples:

- Grade 1 - easily pulled out
- Grade 2 - can be pulled out but will not remain everted
- Grade 3 - may not pull out

It has not been shown that any method of everting the nipples is effective, including the wearing of breast shells. If the nipple does not pull out into the baby's mouth during feeding, there will be a lack of stimulation to produce more milk and continue lactating. In these cases, the infant can become malnourished and dehydrated.

### Breastfeeding During Pregnancy

Breastfeeding during pregnancy is not harmful to the mother or the fetus. If the mother continues to breastfeed her child on demand, there will be no loss of milk. It has been reported that the taste of the milk may change around the third or fourth month of pregnancy which may encourage some children to wean or nurse less. It is important to make certain that the child is receiving enough nourishment and not losing weight due to a decrease in breastmilk. There may be some discomfort when the nipples become sensitive. Once the baby is born, the mother can tandem nurse. Both the infant and the child can still breastfeed. Tandem nursing appears to deepen the relationship between the children and lessen the older child's feelings of isolation from his or her parents when the new baby arrives.

### Elements of Abusive Relationships

Admission of any of these actions on the part of her partner may indicate abuse:

- Fear of or threats by her partner, worries that her actions cause the abuse.
- Being or nearly being grabbed, punched or physically harmed.
- Hurting or threatening to hurt pets or committing property destruction.
- Threatening home destruction or property confiscation.
- Denial of medication, medical care, or insistence on accompanying her to all medical exams.
- Controlling all financial resources, refusal to pay bills.
- Hiding important documents.
- Threatening harm to or taking away existing children or threatening to harm himself or another loved one.
- Denial of access to social outlets and communication with others.
- Preventing her from going to work or school, or making her feel constantly watched.
- Making her feel devalued or forcing her to have sexual relations that are demeaning or damaging.

If any one of the above conditions is true, the mother should be referred to the National Domestic Abuse Hotline (800) 799- SAVE or (800) 787-3224 (TDD).

### Domestic Violence

Domestic violence is a pattern of behavior that includes threatened or actual violence committed by an intimate partner. It includes physical, emotional, or psychological abuse such as becoming detached or uncaring of loved ones. This behavior seeks to create power for the abusive individual by controlling another's life. The abuse can include personal humiliation, sexual degradation, social isolation and financial dependence upon the abuser. While the abuser may apologize later, the abuse continues. The mother may not interpret these actions as abuse and seek to justify the behavior. Certain cultural or religious backgrounds may play a role in the behavior of both partners. The violence may begin or become worse at pregnancy because it is viewed as a threat. Abuse may result in bleeding, miscarriage, vaginal and cervical infections, high blood pressure, premature labor and fetal distress. The mother may suffer from low weight gain and the fetus from low birth weight.

### Protein, Glucose, and Ketones in Urine

Proteinuria in conjunction with gestational hypertension is a hallmark of preeclampsia. It can also occur due to renal damage suffered in acute pyelonephritis. There are no observable physical anomalies indicating early preeclampsia, the blood pressure and urine must be routinely monitored. Acute pyelonephritis presents with many other physical symptoms, including fever, hematuria, myalgia, cystitis, and CVA tenderness.

The urine is routinely screened for glucose and ketones to monitor for symptoms of diabetes. Glucose is spilled into the urine when lack or ineffectiveness of insulin causes the cells of the body to be unable to up glucose to use for energy. The excess glucose is cleared through the kidneys and excreted in the urine. Ketones are metabolic breakdown products of fat and protein which the cells use for energy in place of the unavailable glucose. Ketones cause acidosis which, in the extreme stages of diabetes, can cause coma and death.

## Dating Pregnancies

The following methods have been used to date pregnancies:

- Basal body temperature charting: coital record, ovulation record and temperature elevations with menstrual history.
  - Accuracy: +/- 2 to 5 days and depends on record keeping capability.
- First trimester ultrasound: range of accuracy of +/- 3 to 5 days.
  - Accuracy: depends on gestational age, sonographer's skill, fetal position, and available technology.
- Serum BhCG of less than 10,000, using two values obtained 1 week apart and rising appropriately.
  - Accuracy +/- 3 to 5 days.
- Last accurately recorded normal, regular menstrual period that is consistent with a first trimester exam.
  - Accuracy +/- 1 to 2 weeks.
- Second trimester ultrasound.
  - Accuracy +/- 1 to 2 weeks depending on the requirements for accurate ultrasound.
- Third trimester ultrasound.
  - Accuracy +/- 2 to 3 weeks, depending on the ultrasound conditions.
- Physical exam after 20 weeks.
  - Accuracy +/- 2 to 3 weeks.

## Gestational Age Equivalencies and Post Date Pregnancy

Gestational age equivalencies refer to the various methods of dating a pregnancy. The most common method is the menstrual age. The pregnancy is dated in reference to the first day of the last normal menstrual period.

The menstrual age, the gestational age and the fetal age are all identical. The average length of pregnancy is 280 days (40 weeks or 10 lunar months/9 calendar months).

Conceptual age and ovulatory age are identical. The average length of pregnancy for the conceptual and ovulatory age is 266 days or 38 weeks (9 lunar/8 calendar months). The average gestational age of a pregnancy allows for estimated birth dates within a 4 week range, 2 weeks on either side of the estimated birth date.

A post date pregnancy is considered to be any accurately dated pregnancy that is more than 294 days, more than 42 weeks, or more than 10 lunar months.

## Accurately Dating a Pregnancy

Gestational age must be accurately assessed in order to determine the appropriate time for screening tests that are performed at specific times of the pregnancy. Without accurate dating the screening may be performed at an inappropriate time which in turn leads to misinterpretation of data, unnecessary treatment, or failure to treat when needed. Gestational age at birth is the best predictor of infant well-being and it is the best method for determining the timing of delivery.

Accurate assessment of gestational age becomes more difficult as the pregnancy continues. There are various methods for obtaining enough data to make an accurate assessment, some of which depend upon the woman keeping accurate records in anticipation of conceiving. Since 70% of all conceptions are unexpected, these methods have the lowest compliance rate but one of the highest accuracy rates when used. Other methods depend on various screening or testing methods rather than record keeping.

### Alternative Methods of Gestational Age

Uterine size correlates with gestational age but measurement of the fundus is not a reliable method of measuring uterine size. Factors that can cause discrepancies in a fundal size assessment:

- bladder distension
- position of the fetus
- the length of the cervix
- maternal build
- fibroids
- uterine abnormalities
- placental location
- amniotic fluid volume
- retroflexion or retroversion of the fetus
- placental location
- examiner experience
- foreknowledge of the last menstrual period

The assessment is typically most accurate between 20 and 30 weeks gestation with a margin of error of up to 3 weeks. Quickening and using the time of uterus at the umbilicus as a benchmark for 20 weeks gestation have significantly wide margins of error as do using signs and symptoms of pregnancy or the date on first noting fetal heart tones by ultrasound or fetoscope.

### Naegele's Rule vs Nichol's Rule

Naegele's Rule calculates the EDD by counting back three months from the last menstrual period (LMP) and adding one week. This calculates 10 lunar months or 40 weeks. Note that Mittendorf's study showed the average length of gestation was 41 weeks and 1 day.

Nichol's Rule calculates the EDD in the following way:

First time mothers with 28 day cycles:

LMP + 12 months – 2 months, 14 days = EDD

Second time or more mothers with 28 day cycles:

LMP + 2 months – 2 months, 18 days = EDD

Cycle time > 28 days:

EDD + (days in cycle – 28 days) = EDD

Cycle time < 28 days:

EDD – (28 days – days in cycle) = EDD

The previous menstrual period (PMP) should also be recorded. If the interval between the PMP and the LMP is considerably shorter than the mother's average cycle length (less than three weeks) it is probable that the LMP was implantation bleeding rather than a true period. The EDD should be recalculated accordingly.

## FHT and Palpation of Fetal Movement

The palpation of fetal movement and the presence of fetal heart tones are *confirmatory* signs of pregnancy. The typical fetal heart rate is 120-160 beats per minute. There is no predictive value in the heart rate for determining the gender of the fetus.

## Location of Fetal Heart Tones

Fetal heart tones should be audible by 20 weeks gestation. The abdomen should be palpated for the presentation, position, lie, and variety prior to auscultation of the fetal heart tones. In order to clearly hear the tones, the position of the convex portion of the fetus must be known in relation to the anterior uterine wall. Once found the position of the heart tones can also confirm the previously determined lie, position and presentation. In a cephalic presentation the fetal heart tones can be heard midway between the umbilicus and the level of anterior superior iliac spine. In a breech presentation with anterior variety, fetal heart tones are heard level with or above the umbilicus. With a breech in transverse variety, the heart tone is near the abdominal midline. With a breech in posterior variety, the heart tones are heard in the flank area or near the midline on the opposite side of the abdomen.

## Fetal Tachycardia

Fetal tachycardia in conjunction with late decelerations or prolonged variable decelerations without variability indicates fetal hypoxia. Meconium may or may not be present. If the fetus is at term and the only issue is tachycardia, it is unlikely that the outcome will be negatively impacted. A premature fetus or a post-term fetus, however, is not able to withstand the stresses of the underlying conditions as well as a term fetus. Tachycardia with no other fetal heart rate changes may indicate: hyperthyroidism, fetal anemia, maternal dehydration, congenital anomalies, maternal hyperthermia, fetal hypoxia, administration of drugs such as beta-sympathomimetics, hypertension or asthma medications, and prematurity with gestational age less than 28 weeks. The cause of tachycardia must be identified and treated whenever possible and other tests of fetal well-being should be used such as scalp stimulation or scalp blood sampling.

## Fetal Bradycardia

Fetal bradycardia with a heart rate >80 bpm with appropriate variability rarely indicates acidemia. No variability with prolonged or late decelerations is typically found in hypoxia and metabolic acidosis. Sever hypoxia can present with a bradycardia with no variability and no return to baseline; this condition worsens over time and may be seen immediately before intrauterine fetal death. With bradycardia only, at rates of 100-120 bpm, the following may be present: maternal hypothermia, administration of drugs such as propanolol, prolapsed cord or cord compression, cardiac abnormalities, vagal stimulation, or fetal hypoxemia or asphyxia. With rates of less than 110 bpm an immediate assessment should be performed for a prolapsed cord, expected time until delivery, duration of the bradycardia, the presence/absence of variability, and late or prolonged decelerations. Sustained bradycardia with positive fetal movement is indicative of a complete or incomplete atrioventricular heart blockage.

## Fetal Scalp Stimulation

If assessment of fetal well-being does not give a reassuring result, the fetal scalp can be stimulated in an attempt to increase the heart rate. The fetal scalp can be massaged through the dilated cervix with a finger for 15 seconds. If this does not create the desired response, an Allis clamp may be used to pinch the scalp. The fetal heart rate should accelerate for at least 15 seconds. If electronic fetal monitoring or auscultation is being performed at the time of a pelvic exam, any acceleration during the exam should be recorded as a reassuring sign of wellness. Another method of stimulating the fetal heart rate is through vibroacoustic stimulation. The result is typically a startle, activity, and FHR accelerations. However, if fetus is startled from a sleep state to an awake state tachycardia may result. The fetus must be monitored until a normal baseline heart rate is established.

### Fetal Kick Count

Fetal movement is a reassuring symptom of a healthy pregnancy. Counting and recording the number of movements within a particular period of time each day can help determine if the number of movements is decreasing from a previously determined norm. If there is a significant decrease in movement, there is a high probability of a problem. If movement ceases, fetal death is a significant probability. Cigarette smoking can dramatically depress fetal activity. The methods used are not significant as long as accurate and precise results can be obtained.

Count-to-ten method: One count session is performed at the same time each day. The time taken to reach 10 movements is recorded. At least 10 movements should be felt in 10 hours. If there are fewer than 10 movements, if the time to reach 10 movements is increasing, or if no movement is felt within 10 hours, the woman should contact you.

### Fundal Height

A bimanual exam is used to assess the fundal height:

- 10 weeks: fundus is very slightly above the pubic bone
- 12 weeks: fundus is a few centimeters above the pubis
- 16 weeks: fundus is halfway between the pubic bone and the umbilicus
- 20 weeks: fundus is exactly at the umbilicus, whether single or multiple fetuses, regardless of the size the fetus will attain by term.

If the uterine size does not correlate to the EDD, the menstrual history should be reevaluated.

Mothers may not have an accurate EDD if:

- Their cycle is irregular
- They are breastfeeding and conceive prior to having a period
- They continue to have a period
- They are uncertain of their dates

If the uterus does not seem large enough at the time of the second prenatal visit, a pregnancy test should be performed prior to continuing the exam.

### Fundal Height

Fundal height is determined starting about 22 to 24 weeks of gestation and serves to measure progressive growth and size for dates. If the height does not increase over a period of time perform an investigation into intrauterine growth restriction or fetal death. Inappropriate height for dates also indicates problems.

The least used and most accurate method after 22 to 24 weeks gestation uses calipers to measure the length between the superior border of the symphysis pubis and the top of the fundus. The second most accurate, and the most popular, method relies on a tape measure. The zero line of the tape is placed on the superior border of the symphysis pubis and the tape stretched along the midline of the abdomen to the top of the fundus. The number of centimeters should approximately equal the number of gestational weeks. All healthcare workers measuring the fundal height should notate the method used or try to standardize to one method.

## Fundal Height Using Gross Approximations

The least accurate method is measured with the examiner's fingerbreadths and depends on the position of fundal height in relation to the symphysis pubis, umbilicus, and tip of the xyphoid process at various weeks of gestation. It can be a rough guide when calipers or measuring tapes are not available. Another method uses a tape measure with the zero line on the superior border of the symphysis pubis. Hold the tape between the index and middle finger with the edge of the little finger on the top of the fundus. The measurement is the number of centimeters where the tape meets the fingers plus additional centimeters depending on the fundal relationship to the umbilicus.

## Leopold's Maneuvers 1 and 2

Leopold's Maneuvers indicate fetal lie, presentation, position or variety. It is typically performed at or around 36 weeks. There are four maneuvers starting from the top of the fundus. The palmar flat of the fingers are used for palpating and just enough pressure is used to obtain accurate readings. The first three maneuvers are performed while standing to one side of the mother and facing her head.

In the first maneuver, the top of the fundus is palpated with one hand on either side of the fundus. This maneuver identifies whether the lie is longitudinal or transverse and whether the fetus is in breech.

The second maneuver is midway between the fundus and symphysis pubis. The area from the abdominal midline to the lateral side and from the symphysis pubis to the fundus is palpated by holding the fetus to one side and palpating with the other, then reversing. This will indicate the variety and the position: anterior, posterior, or lateral.

## Leopold's Maneuvers 3 and 4

The third maneuver consists of grasping the lower abdomen immediately above the symphysis pubis between the thumb and middle finger of one hand. Findings from the first and third maneuvers should be compared to make a definitive determination of the lie and presentation. The fourth maneuver is done facing the mother's feet. The bottom of the fundus is palpated with both hands. This will determine presentation and engagement.

## Estimating Fetal Weight

Determining the estimated fetal weight (EFW) demands a great deal of practice and experience to become accurate enough for the measurement to be useful. There is no precise tool at this time to accurately measure the EFW for comparison. The EFW is important during the intrapartal period to determine adequacy of the maternal pelvis for the fetal size. Prenatally, the EFW is one of the measurements used to determine gestational age and progressive fetal growth. This method of estimating the fetal weight can be used in conjunction with ultrasound to develop more accurate readings in the field. Accuracy is best with the midrange of fetal size but becomes more inaccurate for smaller or larger fetuses. One way to practice and become more accurate is by palpating as many mothers as possible in a labor and delivery unit and comparing the EFW with the actual birthweight of the baby.

## Lie, Presentation, Position and Variety of the Fetus

Before 20 weeks of gestation it is unlikely that the lie, presentation, position or variety of the fetus can be felt due to uterine size, toughness, and the high ratio of amniotic fluid to fetal mass in the amniotic sac. Not until the 36th week will any of these factors come into play. At this point, the fetus is generally settled into its intrapartal position although it is possible it may turn again. Perform Leopold's maneuvers of abdominal examination by palpation for the lie, presentation, position or variety. Malpresentation prior to 36 weeks is not significant. However, after 36 weeks, malpresentation may require intervention. The midwife should determine at the very beginning of labor whether the malpresentation still exists as part of management planning for this period.

## Pregnancy Diet

A well balanced diet includes foods from all food groups in prescribed amounts. This ensures proper nutrition by allowing the mother to obtain all required nutrients from food. If a mother takes in 80-100 grams of protein, salt to taste, and water to thirst, in addition to eating the appropriate amount of all food groups, she will be more likely to deliver a healthy baby with no nutritionally oriented birth defects. The mother should take in:

- 2-3 servings of meat, fish, nuts, legumes, or tofu
- 2-3 servings of dairy
- 2 servings of green vegetables
- 1 serving of yellow vegetables
- 3 servings of fruit
- 3 servings of whole grains
- salt to taste
- 6-8 glasses of water each day

Pre-eclampsia can be prevented by eating at least 75 grams of protein a day. Adequate folic acid prevents neural tube defects such as spina bifida.

## Nutritional Counseling

If the diet history shows a lack of true nutritional elements, begin with praise for any positives of the diet. Suggestions for improvement should be based on the mother's own preferences. A diet that seems lacking in variety may signify a lack of resources to secure better nourishment; she should be referred to public assistance. Qualification for assistance may require a letter from you verifying the pregnancy and stating the risks of inadequate weight gain. She should then be taught to create meals from her own best choices of foods. Do not attempt to replace core foods or ingredients with healthier selections if they are part of an ethnic or regional dietary preference. Other sources for nutritional deficiencies can be found. This is also true of preferences for sweets or other treats. Unrealistic recommendations may cause the mother to become non-compliant and incommunicative about her eating habits. This will hinder any investigation into later concerns or complications.

## Vegan Mothers

A vegan mother may have trouble ingesting enough B-12 which can cause serious anemia and neurological damage to the mother and the fetus. Supplemental B-12 in the active form of cyanocobalamin or hydroxocobalamin is the easiest remedy. Fermented soy products, shiitake mushrooms, seaweed, and spirulina have been offered as sources of B-12 but actually contain an analog of B-12 that can block the actual B-12 from being absorbed. Fortified soy products or fresh juices are good sources of B-12 as are sublingual tablets.

## Mothers Who Prefer Organic Foods

Mothers who eat organic foods generally are healthier looking than those who eat more highly processed food. Quality in food choices counts as well as how the food is selected and when it is eaten. Mothers who do not have addictions to sugar, caffeine, alcohol, or marijuana can trust their instincts about food, even when it seems they are craving one food above others.

## Fetal Brain and Organ Development

Brain growth consists of hyperplasia and hypertrophy of cell growth. Malnutrition decreases both types of growth and can result in a smaller brain. Malnutrition during hyperplastic cellular growth causes irreversible damage because a reduced number of cells will be created. Improved nutrition during any phase of hypertrophy can increase cell size as needed and reverse any previous damage. Malnutrition retards other organ development as well. The fetal body and organs do not grow as large as when proper nutrition is maintained. This results in low birth weight infants who are small for gestational age. Perinatal mortality, intellectual disability, cerebral palsy, visual, hearing and neurological defects, and poor perinatal growth and development all increase. Poor nutrition is often found in those who use tobacco, alcohol, caffeine, marijuana, cocaine or other illicit drugs. Multiple gestation, lactose intolerance, eating disorders, and strict vegetarianism can also cause malnutrition.

## Physical Changes During Pregnancy

As estrogen, progesterone and relaxin affect the joints, pain may occur, particularly in the pelvic region. Maintaining good posture, even though the growth of the infant in the uterus places the body off balance, will help prevent or relieve some of the typical aches and pains of the skeletal system.

Exercise also benefits the joints, keeping them limber and less likely to stiffen. Various exercises, such as pelvic rocking and other centering activities, help keep the back muscles strong and improve the spinal alignment. Some joint pain may be alleviated by ensuring proper support when sitting or lying down. The side-lying position is best for pregnancy.

Strengthening muscles such as the gluteals, abdominals, hamstrings, and upper back; and stretching others, such as the psoas, low back, and chest, can keep proper skeletal alignment more easily.

## Pigmentation Changes of the Skin

The nipple and primary areola darken in the third month of gestation. Secondary areolae, linea nigra and abdominal striae appear. Striae is also seen on extremely large breasts and sometimes the buttocks and upper thighs. Chloasma, or mask of pregnancy, may appear.

Pigment changes may be caused by estrogen or progesterone stimulating the melanocytes of the skin. The linea nigra appears as a dark line from the umbilicus to the symphysis pubis at the abdominal midline. Nipple pigmentation varies with complexion; blondes have pink nipples and brunettes have brown nipples. Chloasma is most prevalently seen in brunettes. Sometimes pigment changes will not be seen in pregnancy and occasionally certain pigment changes can be seen in non-pregnant women taking hormones or who may have tumors in other areas.

## Issues of Pregnancy

All of these conditions are primarily attributed to hormonal changes. Nausea and vomiting affect approximately 50% of pregnancies. Small frequent meals are recommended to keep the blood sugar stable. It is thought that psychological and neurological adjustments may be the causes. A small percentage develops hyperemesis gravidarium in which vomiting becomes excessive and self-perpetuating which requires referral to a physician.

During pregnancy the breasts become tender and slightly larger; the areola color deepens and the nipples enlarge. There are usually no serious issues.

Headache is a common complaint during pregnancy. Fatigue, sinusitis and other issues may increase the frequency and severity of headaches. If the headaches occur in the third trimester along with increased blood pressure and/or proteinuria, refer for immediate medical attention.

Fatigue occurs in the first and third trimesters and postnatally. It is caused by bodily changes, then to labor and infant care. There is usually no serious issue.

### Remedies for Sleeping Difficulties

Sleeping difficulties due to pregnancy can be relieved by several methods:

- Deep relaxation and healthy exercise during the day will create proper physical conditions for sleep.
- A silken eye pillow filled with flax seed and lavender may help.
- Stronger remedies can be used if needed; half a dropperful of Skullcap tincture or Valerian tincture may be beneficial.
- In the last trimester, half a dropperful of Hops tincture can help.
- If anxiety and worry are keeping sleep at bay, homeopathic Aconite 30C can be an effective calming agent but should only be used during episodes of anxiety.
- Lemon balm and oats/oat straw have been found to be calming as well.

### Morning Sickness

Morning sickness is caused by elevated estrogen and hCG levels. It is most likely to occur when the stomach is empty but may also occur due to cooking odors. Stress can cause morning sickness to worsen, making emotional support networks and stress reduction essential. In addition, 50mg of Vitamin B-6 at bedtime and midday can also lessen the feelings of nausea. Other ways to reduce the queasy feeling are to eat crackers or plain yogurt when rising in the morning and to drink ginger or raspberry leaf tea. Small meals and keeping food in the stomach may help since morning sickness can be caused by low blood sugar. If vomiting occurs, ground ginger capsules with meals and daily contact with the midwife is advisable, even if only by phone. In the event hyperemesis gravidarium develops severe dehydration may result, requiring an immediate visit to the consulting physician.

### Sciatica

Sciatica is a pain that runs along the sciatic nerve, a large nerve extending from the lower back and down the back of each leg. The pain is felt in the buttocks and leg and becomes worse when sitting. Sometimes the leg or foot can become weak or numb. The pain can be constant on one side of the buttocks and the pain may become shooting when attempting to stand. Often it only affects one side of the lower body. Pregnancy is only one cause of sciatica. It may result from the pressure of the uterus on the sciatic nerve or from muscular tension or vertebral compression from the extra weight and posture changes in pregnancy. Treatment aims to relieve pressure and inflammation. Medications such as non-steroidal anti-inflammatories are used to relieve inflammation while physical therapy can relieve both inflammation and pressure.

### PRURITUS (SKIN ITCHINESS)

pruritus may manifest due to a compromised liver from liver disease, excessive alcohol or recreational drugs, or prolonged use of other medications. It occurs in 3-14% of mothers. Liver tonics of dandelion root and yellow dock root can be effective in reducing the itch. Beets, dark greens, lemon juice and olive oil have liver-cleansing properties as are choline-rich foods like egg yolk, wheat germ, and brewer's yeast. Topical treatments can include plain yogurt rubbed into the skin or oatmeal baths. Itchiness in the palms of the hands or soles of the feet can indicate intrahepatic cholestasis. While this is rare in the general population, it is common in women of Chilean, Mediterranean, or Scandinavian descent. A consult with a backup physician is advisable to determine the need for a liver profile.

### PEMPHIGOID GESTATIONIS (HERPES GESTATIONIS)

Pemphigoid gestationis is a skin condition that is of unknown etiology but may begin with a maternal autoimmune response to paternal antigens that is prolonged by pregnancy hormones. It typically begins in the second trimester and can extend to the postpartum period. The primary complaint is generalized itching and burning of the skin and an erythematous rash. The rash begins on the abdomen and spreads to the rest of the trunk and to the extremities. Blisters develop that can subsequently become infected. Once the diagnosis is confirmed by skin biopsy, topical or oral steroids may be prescribed. Labor is often induced in the $37^{th}$ week due to placental insufficiency and growth restriction. The baby may be born with a slight rash. The mother's lesions will heal after birth but may take several years with periodic resurgence at menstruation, ovulation, or when taking oral birth control medication. It may also recur in future pregnancies, especially those with the same partner.

### YEAST INFECTIONS IN PREGNANCY

Yeast infections, also called monilia, are common during pregnancy. It causes a white, curdish discharge with a yeasty odor. Yeast is part of the normal flora of the vagina that overgrows due to the higher alkalinity of the vaginal secretions during pregnancy and the associated increase in progesterone levels. It can increase the risk of newborn thrush if present at birth. Yeast overgrowth can be controlled with the insertion of vaginal sponges (boiled to remove mineral deposits) or cotton tampons which have been soaked in acidophilus culture solution. The lightly squeezed, saturated sponge or tampon is inserted into the vagina and changed every three hours. Cotton underwear should be worn.

### BACTERIAL VAGINOSIS

Bacterial Vaginosis (BV) is a common vaginal infection. It is also known as gardnerella or hemophilus. It can cause chorioamnionitis, premature rupture of the membranes, and preterm labor when it presents during pregnancy. Indications include:

- A fishy odor to the vaginal secretions, especially after sexual intimacy.
- Thin, gray or white discharge that adheres to the vaginal walls.
- Typically no vaginal irritation or itching.

Diagnosis is made with the Whiff test in conjunction with the symptomology. A cotton swab saturated with vaginal discharge is touched to KOH (potassium hydroxide) solution. If a potent fishy odor, caused by amines, is released, the diagnosis is BV. Insert a garlic clove, peeled and without nicks, into the vagina to be changed three times a day, followed by five days of acidophilus treatment. If unresolved, medical treatment is indicated. The parents should abstain from sexual intimacy and the partner may need to be investigated as well.

## Anemia

Normal hemoglobin in a menstruating woman is 12.0 g/dl and in a pregnant woman is 11.0 g/dl due to an increase in plasma rather than a decrease in red blood cells. A complete blood count (CBC) will help differentiate the cause of any anemia. A hemoglobin level below 10.0 g/dl is cause for concern.

Signs of significant anemia:

- pallor
- jaundice
- tachypnea or dyspnea on exertion
- splenomegaly
- tachycardia or flow murmur
- orthostatic hypotension
- peripheral edema
- smooth and sore tongue
- pale mucus membranes and nail beds

Symptoms:

- poor appetite or changes in food preferences
- changes in mood
- changes in sleep habits
- pica
- malaise
- headaches
- weakness
- dizziness
- fatigue
- drowsiness

95% of pregnancy related anemia is iron deficiency anemia, but a history of any hematologic abnormalities should be investigated.

## Indigestion or Heartburn

During pregnancy the stomach and intestines are displaced by increasing uterine size, especially during the third trimester, causing gastric reflux. In addition, the gall bladder is not as efficient in pregnancy. Frequent small meals and digestive aids seem to be the most effective remedy. Limiting fat intake can decrease issues due to gall bladder insufficiency. Meals should be completed well before lying down at night as food in the stomach when the mother is supine exacerbates heartburn. Some effective digestive aids are Dandelion Leaf or Red Raspberry leaf in herbal infusions or other ingestion method, and Slippery Elm lozenges, which work for extreme heartburn. Raw almonds, raw papaya, or papaya enzyme tablets can also help relieve heartburn and aid digestion.

## Constipation During Pregnancy

Constipation is a common issue during pregnancy. It can be avoided by maintaining proper hydration and eating a diet rich in fiber. Fiber can also help to resolve constipation once it begins. Intestinal motility is reduced in pregnancy allowing for greater water reabsorption from the gut, as well as intestinal compression and ingestion of iron supplements can be causes of constipation.

Persistent constipation can lead to hemorrhoids which can in turn cause difficulties during birth. You should be certain to monitor bowel habits during the course of the pregnancy and offer measures such as those above to alleviate the problem and manage it to avoid the bleeding and discomfort of hemorrhoids.

## Constipation

Compression of the lower intestine due to the increasing weight and size of the uterus contributes to constipation. It is also possible that hormonal changes slow the motility of the intestinal tract causing increased water absorption from the contents of the gut, thereby causing constipation. Oral iron therapy can exacerbate the condition. Ingesting fiber and maintaining hydration, and getting the recommended exercise helps alleviate most problems of this sort. If additional fiber is needed, psyllium seed (the main ingredient of Metamucil) can be taken as a capsule or mixed into food with plenty of water to drink. Prune juice is also very effective. If constipation is not relieved, hemorrhoids may develop which can contribute to difficulties during birth. They can become very painful and may bleed. Avoidance of hemorrhoids should be the basic aim of constipation relief although a secondary effect is the comfort of the mother.

## Migraines

Migraines tend to be seen in adolescents, early adulthood, through middle age. They are often unilateral, severe and cause throbbing pain, nausea and vomiting, and sensitivity to light or noise. Prior to the migraine striking, there are often recognizable symptoms of its approach which can last for days prior to the migraine (prodromes). The most common symptoms are light and noise sensitivity, irritability, mood changes, drowsiness, and increased thirst and hunger. Some may experience aura an hour prior to the migraine. Migraines may be avoided by changes of lifestyle and avoiding known causes of the migraines. Severity and frequency determine medication type and frequency. Mild, infrequent migraines may only need NSAIDs, acetaminophen or aspirin. Tryptans, tricyclic antidepressants, and ergotamine preparations may be used for more severe attacks although these are contraindicated for pregnancy. Pregnancy can cause migraines in those who never suffered them before. Menstrual migraines may be controlled by stabilizing the estrogen levels with birth control pills.

## Causes of Headaches

The most common headaches are migraines and tension headaches. Less common are headaches caused by:

- infections
- cerebrovascular events
- meningitis
- tumors
- glaucoma
- dental issues
- overuse of medication
- arteriovenous abnormalities

Immediately refer any sudden, severe headache that persists despite remedies to a neurologist. If the patient is over 40 and the headache is a new complaint, it may be due to a tumor and she should be referred to a physician. If it is referred to as the worst headache the patient ever had, there is the possibility of hemorrhage into the brain and the patient should be immediately evaluated by a physician. A thorough history to investigate headache issues should include a full description of the headache, frequency and onset, location, precipitating factors if known, family trends, menstrual history, and any other conditions such as neck stiffness, visual complaints, and head trauma.

### Tension Headaches

Tension headaches can be chronic or episodic. They tend to begin in early adulthood and are more common in women than men. Episodic headaches are rarely reported for treatment. Chronic headaches may last for hours with a high frequency. While women with chronic headaches suffer diminished function. They are also more likely to have mood disorders or anxiety. Lifestyle changes that include relaxation techniques and stress reduction plus validation of the issue can help decrease the severity of these headaches. Medications such as acetaminophen or NSAIDs may be ineffective. A combination of 400 mg ibuprofen and 200 mg caffeine has proven more effective than either alone. A combination of behavioral therapy for stress management and tricyclic antidepressants also proved more effective than either alone.

### Backache, Ligament Pain and Leg Cramps

Backache is common in all trimesters of pregnancy due to the growing uterus and its effect on the posture. Relaxin also impacts the ligaments creating backache. Using proper posture and lifting techniques and avoiding standing for long periods can decrease the discomfort. Pelvic tilts, walking, swimming and a supportive maternity girdle can also ease backache pain.

Ligaments stretch under the influence of Relaxin. As the uterus grows and stretches the supporting ligaments, sharp spasms called ligament pain occur. Warm baths, massage, and avoiding stretching can relieve the symptoms.

Leg cramps tend to occur during the third trimester. The cramping may be caused by lowered serum ionized calcium and increased phosphates. Leg stretches before bed and a decrease in the intake of milk, carbonated soft drinks and processed foods may decrease the frequency of cramps. When a cramp occurs, the mother should flex the foot in the opposite direction of the cramp.

### Edema and Varicosities

Edema is a common complaint in pregnancy. Edema of the ankles is a typical issue. It is often exacerbated by activity or hot weather. Edema of the upper shins, breastbone or sacrum is definitive for hemoconcentration. When coupled with proteinuria and/or hypertension it is indicative of preeclampsia and should be investigated and treated immediately. The degree of edema can be assessed by observing for pitting, or observing if an indentation in the edematous tissue remains.

The degree of edema is rated by depression size:

$$+1 = 2\text{mm}$$
$$+2 = 4\text{mm}$$
$$+3 = 6\text{mm}$$
$$+4 = 8\text{mm}$$

Any pitting of +2 or higher is indicative of preeclampsia.

Varicosities tend to occur in pregnancy in those predisposed to them. They may be predictive of deep vein thrombosis. Varicosities can cause pain and reddened or white areas on the calf, secondary to deep vein thrombosis or phlebitis. Referral to a physician is recommended.

## Varicosities During Pregnancy

Genetic predisposition may play one role in the tendency of a woman to develop varicose veins during pregnancy. The pressure of the enlarged uterus on the pelvic veins when the mother is sitting or standing can create poor venous circulation and increase venous pressure on the legs. This can also impact the vena cava when she is lying down. Constrictive clothing can exacerbate the problem as can standing for long periods of time. Smooth muscle relaxation caused by progesterone adds to the issue as well by impacting the venous walls and valves. Remedies include the use of support hose, elasticized sport wraps, or elastic stockings. These should be applied to the legs after the legs have been elevated and also before rising from bed in the morning. Rest with the legs elevated throughout the day, decreased standing time, avoidance of crossing the legs and constrictive clothing will help mitigate the problem.

## Foot and Leg Exercises

Since circulation is not as efficient in pregnancy, especially venous return, cramping, varicose veins, and edema can occur easily. Circulation can be improved by moving the feet and legs on a regular basis, avoiding standing or crossing the legs, and by putting the feet up several times a day. The mother should sit with the legs supported. The ankles are bent and stretched at least 12 times. Both feet are circled at the ankle at least 20 times each direction. Then both knees are braced and held for a count of 4. The legs are then relaxed. This final exercise should be repeated 12 times. For the most effectiveness, these exercises should be done before getting up from bed, at night just before bed and several times a day.

## Dyspareunia

Dyspareunia is defined as pain during sexual intercourse. The pain may be caused by pelvic/vaginal congestion from impaired circulation by uterine pressure. The abdominal enlargement may cause positional changes that are painful. Psychological causes may occur from misconceptions about sex during pregnancy and fear of harming the fetus. Positional changes may alleviate some issues due to an enlarged abdomen and ice may reduce congestion but cause its own discomfort. Discussion of any fears regarding sexual intercourse may alleviate psychological issues. Alternative sexual practices may be recommended.

## Transverses Exercise and Pelvic Tilting

The transverse exercise tones the deep transverse abdominal muscles and helps prevent backache due to poor posture. Sit or kneel on hands and knees with a level spine. Breathe in then release. Pull in the lower part of the abdomen below the umbilicus without moving the spine and continue to breathing normally. Hold the muscles for 10 seconds then gently relax. Repeat up to 10 times.

The pelvic tilt or rocking exercise is performed in a half-sitting position with plenty of support from pillows. Bend the knees and place the feet flat on the floor. Place one hand under the small of the back and the other on the abdomen. Tighten the abdominal and the buttocks and press the small of the back into the floor. Breathe normally. Hold this position for 10 seconds and release. Repeat up to 10 times.

## Bleeding or Spotting During Pregnancy

Any spotting or bleeding is cause for concern. If there is non-rhythmic pain, a tubal pregnancy may be suspected. Persistent bleeding implicates a missed abortion or (rarely) molar pregnancy. Other causes of bleeding:

- severe cervicitis
- cervical lesions

- cervical polyps
- subchorionic bleeding
- post-coital bleeding
- implantation spotting
- fetal death of a twin without expulsion of the tissue

Placental problems cause chronic bleeding late in pregnancy.

Cervical bleeding is caused by infections, such as gonorrhea, chlamydia, Trichomonas, or cervical dysplasia. A herpes lesion or a vaginal yeast infection can cause the cervix to be friable. Treatment consists of rest. Sexual intercourse, insertion of anything into the vagina, or engaging in behavior that causes orgasm should not be attempted. Continue to monitor. If the bleeding worsens or is accompanied by pain, refer the mother to a physician.

## First Trimester Bleeding

A thorough history can be an important tool in the differential diagnosis of vaginal bleeding. It should have:

- confirmation of date of the LMP
- any contraceptive use prior to conception, especially IUD use
- results of pregnancy tests
- history of the bleeding: when it started, heaviness, color of the blood and frequency of pad changes
- pain or cramping, when it started and where it is located, severity and intensity
- possibility of recent UTI or STD
- changes in pregnancy symptoms
- whether recent intercourse has occurred

### *Symptoms and General Causes of Vaginal Bleeding During the First Trimester*

One-third of women experiencing first trimester bleeding may be suffering symptoms of abortion. Demise of a twin without expelling products of conception can cause vaginal bleeding. Other causes of first trimester bleeding include:

- ectopic pregnancy
- cervical lesions or polyps
- post-coital bleeding
- implantation spotting
- severe cervicitis
- subchorionic bleed

Any bleeding during the first trimester may endanger the mother or fetus and must be investigated. If the bleeding is light and there is no attendant low abdominal or back pain, the woman should observe precautionary instructions: bodily rest, pelvic rest, avoid orgasm, and notify you of any increase in vaginal bleeding, lower abdominal cramps or backache, pelvic pain, a gush of fluid or fever. Bodily rest does not mean bed rest, only an awareness of symptoms. Sexual intercourse or insertion of any object into the vagina should be avoided except a progesterone suppository if being used.

### *Office Exam in Diagnosing First Trimester Bleeding*

Check the mother's blood pressure, temperature, pulse and respiration and repeat a pregnancy test to confirm pregnancy.

The following should be performed:

- palpation for pain/tenderness, fundal height and masses, rebound tenderness, CVA tenderness, bowel sounds
- a speculum exam for vaginitis, cervicitis, dilations of cervical os, presence in os of any unexpected condition
- a bimanual exam for uterine size, masses, cervical effacement or dilation;
- auscultation of fetal heart tones
- a sonogram, a hemoglobin/hematocrit, and serial quantitative serum BhCG measurements or progesterone measurements

## Cervical and Vaginal Causes of Bleeding

The cervix is extremely vascular in the first trimester. Any inflammation of the tissue can cause bleeding. It is important to examine for the source of the bleeding. If the blood is coming from within the uterus, a sonogram and bloodwork for BhCG and progesterone should be obtained. If the blood is from the cervix itself, it is rarely implicated in pregnancy loss but must still be treated. Infection is a primary cause of cervical bleeding, such as gonorrhea, chlamydia, or trichomonas. Cervical dysplasia may also be at fault. Herpes lesions, yeast infections, polyps, and bacterial vaginosis can also cause cervical bleeding as can sexual intercourse due to increased cervical vascularity. If there is a concern about ectopic pregnancy, a history of repeated miscarriage, or a non-reassuring bimanual exam perform an ultrasound exam.

## Gestational Hypertension

Gestational hypertension, also known as pregnancy induced hypertension, is defined by blood pressure readings of 140/90 or above in repeated readings at least 6 hours apart to rule out readings affected by tension and emotional issues. Readings done with the mother on her left side are thought to be most accurate. Treatment to reduce this type of hypertension includes aerobic exercise, deep relaxation practice, elimination of stimulating foods and drinks and strong spices, a proper diet and herbal supplements, and counseling by a therapist. If readings of 160/100 or more occur, medical intervention is needed.

If blood pressure suddenly increases near term with no other symptoms, it will likely resolve when labor begins. If all else shows readiness for labor, attempt inducing labor. If the blood pressure readings steadily rise during labor, preeclampsia or vascular damage may be beginning. Transport the mother to the hospital.

## Nutrition and Hydration in Pregnancy-Induced Hypertension

Exercise and nutrition, while important in general for pregnancy, can help alleviate pregnancy-induced hypertension. Aerobic exercise increases circulation and dilates blood vessels. If the mother's blood pressure rises to 140/90, rest should be recommended over exercise. Abnormal weight gain, which can be the result of poor nutritional habits, can exacerbate a tendency for high blood pressure but stressing the system. High quality protein, whole grains, and mineral-rich vegetables and fruits should be consumed. Some foods are particularly suited to reduce blood pressure such as watermelon, cucumber, parsley, onion, and garlic. Salt intake should continue according to taste. The consumption of stimulants such as caffeine, nicotine, and cocaine can cause vasoconstriction and low birth weight and should be completely removed from the diet. Strong spices such as mustard, ginger, nutmeg and black pepper may also cause issues and should be reduced or avoided. Fluid intake should be increased.

## Herbal Remedies for Gestational Hypertension

The regular ingestion of Raspberry leaf or Nettle infusions help prevent hypertension. When hypertension occurs, hops, skullcap, passionflower, hawthorn, and chamomile all induce relaxation and reduce systolic pressure. Diastolic pressure can be reduced through the use of cayenne pepper, which acts as a vasodilator and cardiac stimulant. Hops is the most potent of the listed herbs and can be taken nightly as a tea in the last months of pregnancy; but it is contraindicated for regular use throughout pregnancy or for use in the first trimester. Skullcap can be taken as an infusion once or twice daily. Passionflower can be taken in capsule form, 2 to 4 capsules daily, or in tincture at the rate of 15 drops three times daily. Hawthorn is a strong vasodilator that works cumulatively. A cold infusion taken in sips at the rate of one cup daily, or 15 drops of the tincture two to three times a day is recommended.

## Calcium and Magnesium in Hypertension Treatment

The role of calcium in controlling hypertension has not been satisfactorily proven or explained. While studies have shown magnesium and phosphorus intake can impact blood pressure, calcium has not been shown to have the same effect. However, since calcium intake is usually below the recommended levels, ensuring adequate intake during pregnancy is not harmful. Calcium uptake by the body requires adequate magnesium, phosphorus, and Vitamins A, C, and D. The best nutritional sources for calcium are in fish and dairy products. Salmon, sardines, mackerel, seaweed (kelp), sesame salt, tahini, and dark leafy vegetables such as turnip tops, kale and beet greens are all good sources of calcium in food. Nettle and Raspberry leaf infusions both carry calcium and the supporting vitamins and minerals. Many wild greens such as Lamb's Quarters, Mallow, Galinsoga, Shepherd's Purse, Knotweed, Bidens, Amaranth, and Dandelion leaves are good sources of calcium.

## Pregnancy Induced Hypertension

Hypertension is managed according to its severity. Close monitoring is required in the event it progresses into preeclampsia. Rest, appropriate nutrition, and adequate hydration are required. The weight will be monitored along with other parameters. The blood pressure is monitored at home on a daily basis, and every 4 hours if the mother is an inpatient. A daily abdominal exam is performed to identify any tenderness that could signal placental abruption or HELLP syndrome. A biophysical profile is performed to assess fetal well-being. A complete blood count (CBC), coagulation profile, electrolytes, BUN, creatinine, albumin and liver function tests are performed. In severe preeclampsia the blood tests may be repeated every 12 to 24 hours. Certain drugs, such as methyldopa, atenolol, labetalol, and nifedipine may be prescribed as a short-term prophylaxis. Some antithrombolytic agents are also prescribed to prevent DIC and other conditions found in preeclampsia.

## Stress Reduction for Working Mothers

Interview the mother to determine her ability, methods, and time for rest and relaxation during pregnancy. Non-allopathic treatments using Vitamins B and C, calcium, protein and trace minerals, as well as herbal tinctures of hawthorn, passionflower, or hops can help ease chronic stress that can be the proximal cause of night-time pain and insomnia. Chiropractic treatments, massage, deep relaxation and aerobic exercise also help with stress. Advocate resting as soon as work is done, enlisting significant others and family members for support. Quitting work one to two weeks prior to the EDD is essential to prevent an overdue birth. Enough time must be taken from work after the birth to establish bonding, milk supply and a routine. Support of a post-partum doula or other helper and from associations such as the La Leche League will increase the success of the first few weeks. If the mother is a student, discuss a reasonable schedule of classes and homework to enable both the mother and baby to be adequately cared for.

## Hypertension, Phenylketonuria, or Advanced Maternal Age

Chronic hypertension rarely impacts pregnancy as long as blood pressure is under control and the use of ACE inhibitors (FDA Pregnancy Category C) and angiotensin II receptor agonists (FDA Pregnancy Category D), is avoided. Counseling about the risk of preeclampsia and intrauterine growth restriction must be offered.

Phenylketonurics should be counseled to return to dietary therapy prior to conception and strict maintenance of that diet throughout the pregnancy. If the dietary plan is not followed there is a substantial risk of intellectual disability and microcephaly due to exposure in utero to high levels of phenylketones in the mother's system.

Advanced maternal age is defined as delaying conception past the age of 35. There is an increased risk of genetic disorders, gestational diabetes, hypertension and other chronic conditions. Another issue is decreased fertility. You may wish to facilitate a discussion about the changes in lifestyle that occur with bearing and raising children.

## Pre-Eclampsia

Pre-eclampsia occurs in about 5% of pregnancies and tends to start between 20 weeks of gestation and the first week after birth.

Symptoms include:

- Increased blood pressure
- Proteinuria
- Persistent headaches, Blurred vision or sensitivity to light
- Abdominal pain

Pre-eclampsia can lead to placental abruption and can affect the mother's liver, kidneys and brain. It is a leading cause of fetal complications including low birth weight, premature birth, and stillbirth. Mothers at risk for pre-eclampsia include those who have or develop:

- Chronic hypertension
- High blood pressure during a previous pregnancy
- Obesity prior to pregnancy
- An age under 20 years or over 40 years
- Pregnancy with multiple fetuses
- Diabetes
- Kidney disease
- Rheumatoid arthritis
- Lupus
- Scleroderma

There is no cure except to have the baby. Those exhibiting signs of pre-eclampsia must be monitored closely to prevent fetal or maternal damage or death. A home birth is not recommended.

## Pregnancy of a Diabetic Mother

Preconception counseling should be undertaken for diabetic women. Persistent high blood sugar during the first 6 weeks of pregnancy can increase the risk of major congenital abnormalities and/or low birthweight. Educate such women about these risks and create a management plan that includes focusing on maintaining blood sugar level control. If the woman is diet controlled or on oral medication, she may be required to use insulin during the pregnancy. She should be referred to either an obstetrician who specializes in high risk pregnancies or an endocrinologist to help manage the diabetes during her pregnancy. Perform a health assessment focusing on conditions that are high risk in diabetics such as diabetic retinopathy, nephropathy, coronary artery disease (CAD), and hypertension. A history of gestational diabetes in previous pregnancies can increase the risk for developing it in future pregnancies. A management plan that includes a good diet and exercise may reduce the risk of gestational diabetes and/or its complications.

## Cardiac Disease in Pregnancy

Women with cardiac disease should be strongly urged to consult both a cardiologist and obstetrician when planning or managing a pregnancy. The cardiac condition must be thoroughly assessed and the parents educated about the risks involved. The risk is based on: the cardiac lesion, the baseline functional compromise, and the possibilities of complications during pregnancy. Genetic counseling may also be indicated if a condition is the result of inherited heart disease. A decision to terminate the pregnancy to save the mother's life may be required. The following cardiac diseases are examples of those carrying a serious risk of maternal mortality during pregnancy:

- Pulmonary hypertension
- Dilated cardiomyopathy
- Marfan's syndrome
- Any uncorrectable cardiac lesion in classes III or IV refractory to medical management

The woman must anticipate multiple office and hospital visits and close management during the pregnancy. Child care, workplace issues, and insurance should all be taken into consideration in the management plan.

## Thyroid Disorders and Infectious Diseases

Both hyperthyroidism and hypothyroidism are associated with congenital fetal anomalies. Therefore it is important that the woman achieve and maintain euthyroid prior to and during the pregnancy. Refer the woman for medical consultation, especially regarding any medication requirements. Both propylthiouracil and methimazole are FDA Category D pregnancy drugs and alternatives should be prescribed. The management plan should include assessment of thyroid levels.

Many infectious diseases can be screened for and vaccinated against if immunity is not found. This is true of rubella, varicella, and hepatitis B which are common childhood vaccinations or are common infections in childhood. Positive titers for Toxoplasmosis and CMV show that there is minimal pregnancy risk while a negative titer shows non-immunity and education about avoidance can be offered. Testing for STD's including HIV can be performed. Negative results three months prior to preconception generally negate the need to repeat them after pregnancy begins.

## Gestational Diabetes

Complications to the fetus of uncontrolled diabetes include macrosomia, polyhydramnios, and pregnancy induced hypertension or preeclampsia. At each visit abdominal palpation should be performed. If the fundal height is greater than expected for dates, polyhydramnios or macrosomia may be to blame. Ultrasound should be used to confirm fetal size and the amniotic fluid index. If both are normal, routine prenatal care continues. If, however, the fetus is large for dates or the amniotic fluid index is abnormal, consult with a physician.

At 34 to 36 weeks, fetal movement counting should commence. If the fetus is the appropriate size, the amniotic fluid is at the appropriate levels, there is no hypertension and no history of stillbirth, the pregnancy can proceed until labor begins naturally. At 40 weeks a biophysical profile should be performed twice a week until birth. If, however, complications occur, or there is a history of stillbirth, labor should be induced at 40 weeks.

### *Management of Gestational Diabetes*

Maintaining an appropriate level of glucose in the bloodstream is the goal of diabetes management. Most mothers can manage diabetes with diet and exercise while others require the assistance of insulin injections. Nutritional therapy begins with a nutritionist or other professional in diabetic management. Education includes determining food exchanges, types of acceptable foods, determining an appropriate number of calories to ingest and in what forms, and meal planning. Additionally, the mother is counseled in monitoring her blood sugar with the finger-stick method and a commercial glucometer although office visit glucose monitoring can be made available if the woman cannot perform the monitoring herself. Fasting blood sugar should be less than 95 mg/dl, 1 hour postprandial blood sugars should be less than 140 mg/dl and 2 hour postprandial blood sugar should be less than 120 mg/dl. The frequency of monitoring should be determined by the mother and the health care worker to maintain consistent glucose values.

## Urinary Tract Infections

Urinary tract infections are common during pregnancy because urinary stasis occurs due to normal hydronephrosis, creating a breeding ground for bacteria. Urinary tract infections during pregnancy are associated with preterm labor, low birth weight, hypertension, preeclampsia, pyelonephritis and maternal anemia without prompt identification and treatment. Those who have sickle cell trait or anemia, diabetes, or a history of UTI are at higher risk of developing infections. The most common bacteria implicated in UTI is *E. coli* which is part of the normal flora of the intestinal tract but can be pathogenic elsewhere. Other UTI-causing bacteria are *Klebsiella*, *Proteus*, *Pseudomonas aeruginosa*, and beta-hemolytic *Streptococcus*. Treatment consists of prescribing the appropriate antibiotic. UTI during pregnancy often lacks symptoms; it is recommended that screening of the urine be performed at the first prenatal visit. The presence of more than 100,000 bacteria of the same species per milliliter of urine indicates infection.

## Asymptomatic Bacteriuria and Cystitis

Asymptomatic bacteriuria has no associated symptoms and can progress into pyelonephritis with complications of pregnancy. Since up to 40% of untreated UTIs can become pyelonephritis, identification and treatment are paramount concerns.

Cystitis is a condition of inflammation of the bladder, typically caused by a bacterial infection. Symptoms include urinary urgency and frequency, dysuria, nocturia, suprapubic pain, and hematuria. Laboratory examination of the urine will show bacteriuria, increased white blood cells, red blood cells, and nitrites. It is not necessary to await identification of the specific pathogen to begin treatment. Prophylaxis can be changed upon identification if the current therapy proves to be inappropriate. Common antibiotics are sulfa drugs (Bactrim), nitrofurantoin (Macrodantin), cephalosporins, and ampicillin or amoxicillin. Sulfa drugs should not be used past 36 weeks, and nitrofurantoin should not be given to women with G6PD. If Group B Streptococcus is identified, treatment should be given prenatally and in labor.

## Small for Dates

A fetus considered small for dates in the first half of pregnancy is often the result of inaccurate dating.

Other causes in early pregnancy:

- missed abortion
- ectopic pregnancy
- a small maternal frame
- inaccurate first measurement
- fetal or chromosomal abnormality
- placental pathology
- fetal death
- oligohydramnios
- fetal infection
- insufficient intrauterine growth due to maternal illness

Causes in later pregnancy:

- intrauterine growth restriction
- fetal death
- oligohydramnios
- poor maternal weight gain
- transverse or oblique lie
- genetically small infant that is normally grown

Perform an ultrasound to confirm the abdominal examination findings and for differential diagnosis. If needed, give nutritional counseling and assistance to stop smoking and manage any other substance abuse issue. It may be necessary to minimize time in the workplace and reduce stress. If IUGR is diagnosed, contact the consulting physician.

## IUGR

Because a fetus suffering from intrauterine growth restriction (IUGR) has already been stressed from chronic hypoxia, the hypoxic environment during birth will make it more difficult to endure the transition to extrauterine life. Perform supportive care and close monitoring from the onset of labor.

After birth, quickly assess the fetus for visible abnormalities or infection and determine the gestational age. Infant glycogen stores are extremely limited and the infant may suffer from immediate hypoglycemia and hypothermia. Encourage early feedings and screen the infant's blood sugar until it reaches at least 36 mg/dl if the infant is asymptomatic and 45mg/dl if it is symptomatic. Frequent temperature assessments will be required as some infants will not be able to stabilize without an external heat source. Save the placenta and cord blood for examination.

### *Signs and Categorization of Intrauterine Growth Restriction*

If the birthweight of a newborn is below the $10^{th}$ percentile for gestational age, it is considered to be small for gestational age (SGA). The majority have an underlying cause for intrauterine growth restriction (IUGR). Other signs of IUGR are subcutaneous tissue wasting, prominent eyes and firm skulls. There may be compensatory polycythemia. There are two categories of IUGR.

*Symmetrical IUGR* includes infants who were affected early in gestation. They will have both reduced cranial circumference and reduced birthweight. Symmetrical IUGR can be caused by chromosomal anomalies, exposure to drugs or other teratogens, or perinatal infections.

*Asymmetrical IUGR* includes infants who were affected late in gestation, usually the third trimester. The birth weight is below the 10th percentile but the cranial circumference is above the 10th percentile. It is usually due decreased placental blood flow or oxygenation of the fetus.

## Oligohydramnios

Oligohydramnios is a condition in which there is a lower than normal volume of amniotic fluid. This increases the likelihood of cord compression, fetal distress and hypoxia during labor. Prior to labor this condition significantly increases the chances of fetal mortality due to the increased incidence of intrauterine growth restriction, post maturity syndrome, and congenital anomalies. It can be diagnosed by demonstrating a tightly packed fetus within the uterus and a fundal height that is small for dates. Although amniotic fluid can be increased by hydrating the mother or, more rarely, replacing fluid volume with sterile saline, it is best to quickly diagnose the cause of the condition and treat it. If intrauterine growth restriction is determined a hospital birth is recommended.

## Polyhydramnios

Polyhydramnios is a condition of excess amniotic fluid most commonly occurring with multiple pregnancies, Rh incompatibility, or diabetes. Fetal anomalies may also engender polyhydramnios, especially atresia of the esophagus, hydrocephaly, anencephaly or spina bifida. Generally there will be an elevated fundal height at 28 weeks with a steady increase in height as the pregnancy progresses. It may be difficult to palpate the baby and the heart tones may be muffled.

In order to differentiate polyhydramnios from a thick uterine wall check for fluid thrill by placing a hand on either side of the uterus. A positive thrill indicating polyhydramnios is found when a vibration is felt on one side of the uterus when it is tapped on the opposite side. Ultrasound monitoring should be performed to determine the cause. Uterine dysfunction, placental abruption and post-partum hemorrhage may take place during labor due to uterine hyperdistension. Excess fluid can also cause fetal malpresentation and cord prolapse. A hospital birth is recommended.

## Acute Pyelonephritis

Pyelonephritis is an inflammation of the kidney(s), typically due to a bacterial infection. It is the most common non-obstetrical complication resulting in hospitalization for pregnant women.

Complications:

- preterm labor and delivery
- acute respiratory distress syndrome
- septic shock
- hemolysis leading to anemia

Causes:

- ureter compression by the uterus at the pelvic brim
- decreased bladder tone
- dilation of the renal pelves
- urinary stasis

Symptoms:

- fever
- chills
- suprapubic or lumbar pain
- CVA tenderness
- hematuria
- myalgia
- dysuria
- nausea and vomiting
- a history of asymptomatic bacteriuria or cystitis
- Urinary frequency and urgency

Laboratory results include bacteriuria, hematuria, pyuria, and proteinuria, and an increased white count with a left shift. Refer to the consulting physician. Pyelonephritis requires IV therapy for dehydration and electrolyte imbalance. Antibiotic suppressive therapy is usually maintained until delivery.

## Types of Breech Presentations

A breech presentation is one in which the fetus is longitudinal but not head down. Breech presentation types:

- Frank breech: the fetus is flexed at the hips with the legs against the abdomen and the feet in front of the face. This includes nearly 70% of breech births and is very common in a primagravida.
- Complete breech: the arms and legs are flexed and the fetus is sitting on the cervix.
- Footling breech: one or both feet are presenting through the cervix and into the birth canal. This breech position is very rare.
- Knee breech: even more rare, the presenting part is one knee (through the cervix) or both knees, fetus is kneeling on the cervix.

The fetus can assume six different positions within the uterus: left and right sacroposterior, left and right sacrolateral, and left and right sacroanterior.

## Identifying Breech Presentation Prior to Labor

Ultrasound is the best method of identifying a breech presentation. It provides a clear picture of the position and presentation of the fetus at any given time. Palpation may be used to identify a breech although with difficulty in a primagravida with firm abdominal muscles. Palpation shows a longitudinal lie with a soft presentation. The head can be felt in the fundus and is easily movable unless it is a frank breech and the legs do not allow the head to move as freely. Auscultation of the fetal heart tones are typically heard above the umbilicus in a breech unless the hips have engaged in the pelvic brim. In that case, the heart tones will be lower. X-ray is almost never used to identify breech presentation due to the risk to the fetus but it can provide pelvimetric measurements while showing the presentation.

## Turn Breech Presentation Prior to Labor

There are several methods:

- Postural tilting: The mother must empty her bladder and lie down with hips elevated three times a day for 20 minutes.
- Somersaults in a swimming pool.
- Elephant walking, with the mother walking on hands and feet.
- A baby may be turned by placing a rebozo, or large shawl, at the juncture of the mother's thighs and hips while she is on knees and elbows. The midwife then takes the ends of the rebozo and stands at the mother's head and alternates pulling each end forward, creating a rocking motion. This should be performed for several minutes.

Other alternatives, while not strictly postural, may suffice: playing music through headphones low on the mother's uterus, speaking to the baby from low on the uterus, shining a light into the vagina from between the legs or placing a bag of frozen vegetables near the baby's head all may cause the head to turn downward.

## External Cephalic Version

External cephalic version (ECV) is a method of turning a breech to a cephalic presentation.

Note: this procedure should only be performed by a skilled and experienced practitioner in a facility equipped for emergency delivery. This procedure should not be attempted prior to 37 weeks gestation due to risk that the fetus will revert or that labor will begin.

The amniotic fluid volume, position and engagement of the fetus, and maternal parity all play a role in the success of this procedure. Ultrasound determines the placental position, and position and presentation of the fetus. With the woman in a supine position dislodge the breech from the pelvic brim towards an iliac fossa. With one hand on each end of the fetus, gently force the fetus to perform a forward somersault into the cephalic position. If this is not possible, attempt a backward somersault. If the fetus will not easily turn, discontinue the ECV and try again in a few days. Immediately after the attempt auscultate the fetal heart tones and administer Rhogam if the mother is Rh negative mother, in case of placental separation.

## Complications of ECV

Complications that can occur with ECV include separation of the placenta, rupture of the membranes, and knotting of the umbilical cord. With placental separation pain and bleeding may occur during or after the procedure. Rupture of the membranes can lead to a prolapsed cord since no fetal part is engaged in the pelvic brim. A knotted umbilical cord may be diagnosed if bradycardia suddenly presents and persists. It this occurs, the fetus is turned back to breech position and an emergency caesarian section if performed.

A uterine scar from a previous caesarian section may be a contraindication to ECV for some woman. Absolute contraindications for ECV include a hydrocephalic fetus, multiple pregnancy, oligohydramnios, preeclampsia, ruptured membranes, and any condition that requires the fetus to be delivered by caesarian section.

## Methods for Turning a Breech Presentation

Moxibustion originated in China. A stick of dried mugwort is used as a heat source over the Bladder 67 acupuncture point (the lower outer corner of the small toe). The theory of moxibustion is that adrenocortical output is stimulated and increases the release of lactogens. This, in turn, increases myometrial sensitivity and contractility. The fetal heart rate and fetal movements increase and the fetus turns cephalic on its own. One study showed a success rate of 66% to 87%, a higher success rate than external version. Moxibustion should be performed on both feet two to three times daily until version occurs. It is most effective when the mother is on a slant board.

Homeopathic Pulsitilla 30C can be taken several times a day and may help turn a breech. Swimming or performing handstands while immersed in water may also cause a fetus to turn from a breech presentation.

## Maneuvers in Delivering a Breech

Learn methods of breech delivery as well as possible in the event of unexpected breech delivery where transport or caesarian is not possible.

- Pinard maneuver: for delivering a frank breech. It is a method of manipulating the legs of the fetus. The hips are deflexed, the legs are brought down one at a time and the frank breech is changed into a footling. Use this maneuver when delivery has stalled due to a splinting effect of the fetal legs.
- Mauriceau-Smellie-Veit maneuver: for keeping the head flexed once the shoulders are delivered. Place one hand is placed into the vagina to hold the infant's face; the index finger goes into the mouth and the back of the finger is pressed against the maxilla. This is not to provide traction. The rest of the hand supports the head. Place the other hand at the back of the neck with one finger hooked over each shoulder to provide traction.

## Unexpected Breech Delivery

The fetal position may be incorrectly interpreted during palpation or the fetus may turn breech at the last moment.

- Make the room extremely warm.
- Place the mother in an upright position.
- Instruct the mother not to push until the body is born.
- Once the fetal umbilicus and legs are out ensuring there is no tension in the cord; do not handle the cord.
- Wrap the body and umbilical cord in warmed receiving blankets to delay onset of respiration.
- If a frank or complete breech becomes arrested while birthing the body, gently place the legs into an antero-posterior position so the body can descend.
- Once the shoulders are delivered, place the infant into an occipital-anterior position using the hips to guide the body.
- The baby should be allowed to hang until the nape or jaw line is visible.
- Administer additional support after the head is born to stimulate respiration.

## Multiple Gestation

Determine possible multiple gestation by:

- Auscultation of more than one distinct heart tone
- A history of ovulation-inducing drug treatments
- Severe nausea and vomiting beyond that expected in typical morning sickness
- Uterine size, fundal height, and abdominal girth that is large for dates, especially in the second trimester

- A family history of twins
- Discovery by palpation of three or more large body parts especially in the third trimester

If there is a discrepancy between the estimated gestational age and the uterine size at the first prenatal visit, perform an ultrasound to date the pregnancy and show any multiple fetuses. The discrepancy may not be significant until the second or third prenatal visit if the mother began prenatal care very early in pregnancy.

### Risks of Multiple Gestation

Twin pregnancy is at higher risk than singleton for a number of complications:

- malpresentation
- gestational diabetes
- placenta previa
- stillbirth
- fetal abnormalities
- early pregnancy loss
- IUGR
- premature labor and birth
- preeclampsia
- dysfunctional labor

Managing multiples requires exceptional support from a consulting physician. You should expect a hospital birth. Higher order multiples require physician management (triplets and higher). Determine placental placement and chorionicity of twinning by ultrasound for risk identification and management. Chorionicity refers to whether the twins are monozygotic (from the and management. Chorionicity refers to whether the twins are monozygotic (from the splittinof a single embryo) or dizygotic (from the fertilization and implantation of two ova). Amnionicity indicates whether a single amniotic sac is being shared by the fetuses (monochorionic) or whether two separate amniotic sacs are present (dichorionic). In the case of dichorionicity, there may be a single fused placenta with two cords or two separate placentas.

## VBAC

Vaginal birth after C-section (VBAC) is a controversial subject. In 2004, the American College of Obstetrics and Gynecology released a statement "strongly advising" women and birth centers against attempting VBACs in birth centers because the health risks were too great and recommended all VBACs take place in a hospital. It concluded that women with a previous C-section were at increased risk for complications compared to those with no C-section history. The American Academy of Family Physicians released recommendations in 2005 stating women with a single previous caesarian delivery with a low transverse incision should be offered a trial of labor and not restricted to facilities with surgical teams present due to lack of evidence of improved outcomes. However, some hospitals will not offer VBAC services. You should be aware of the situation in your community and about the complete VBAC recommendations so your can fully inform clients who desire VBAC about the choices and risks in labor and delivery.

### Risks of Uterine Rupture During VBAC

The greatest risk of uterine rupture during VBAC is when the previous caesarian section was performed via a vertical incision of the upper contractile uterine segment. Catastrophic uterine rupture may well result, in which the old incision opens completely, the fetal membranes rupture, part or all of fetus extrudes into the peritoneal cavity, and there is significant hemorrhage.

If the caesarian was performed prior to 28 weeks gestation, especially without labor, it indicates the corpus muscular mass was likely incised regardless of type of incision; the risk of rupture in this case may be significant enough to deny a trial of labor. Labor induction increases the risk of uterine rupture, especially if prostaglandins are used.

Risk of rupture may be related to the previous incision closure. A greater risk is found in single layer of continuous running stitch as opposed to a double layer of interrupted sutures. This information may not be available in the medical record.

## Candidates for VBAC

You must have thorough knowledge about the local legal policies of your community. A thorough history and review of previous medical records is essential for determining whether to attempt VBAC. If the previous caesarian section was via vertical incision in the contractile uterine segment, there is a high risk of uterine rupture. Repeat caesarian without trial of labor is indicated.

In most other cases, a trial of labor may be indicated if the pregnancy and labor are otherwise normal. Prenatal management includes referral to a VBAC course or support group and additional support for those without complete familial support for their decision. During labor, management is the same as normal labor except for increased frequency of fetal heart tone auscultation since the typical first indication of uterine rupture is fetal bradycardia. Check FHR every 15 minutes in the first stage and every 5 minutes in the second. Use labor augmentation cautiously. There is an increased possibility of the placenta implanting over the uterine scar and resulting in placenta accreta.

## Factors of Success for VBAC

VBAC may be more successful with:

- a previous history of VBAC
- spontaneous labor with normal progression
- non-repetition of the reason for the previous caesarian section , such as a breech presentation or preeclampsia

In some instances, a trial of labor may end in a repeat caesarian section if the same reasons for the previous caesarian occur such as:

- failure to progress or cephalopelvic disproportion
- the need to induce or augment labor
- no prior vaginal delivery
- more than one previous caesarian section
- a non-reassuring fetal heart tone early in labor

The operative report and record of the previous labor and surgery should be obtained prior to discussing the possibility of VBAC. The mother will not have the necessary medical information. Placement of the abdominal incision does not indicate the placement of the uterine incision.

## Preterm Labor

Immediately assess a woman who appears to be in preterm labor and notify the consulting physician if assessment shows preterm labor. Take a history that includes:

- the present signs and symptoms
- any sign of urinary tract infection, STDs, vaginitis, cervicitis, viral or bacterial infection
- signs of premature rupture of the membranes (PROM)

Include a physical exam:

- vitals
- evaluation of gestational age, contractions, FHT, CVA tenderness, low back or suprapubic pain
- palpation for multiple gestation, position, presentation, and estimated fetal weight.

Pelvic exam:

- assess vaginitis or cervicitis
- STDs
- bloody show
- meconium
- PROM
- cervical changes
- station

If PROM is diagnosed, a digital exam is contraindicated. Laboratory tests should include urine microscopy, urine culture, wet mount for bacterial vaginosis and trichomonas, cultures for Group B Streptococcus, genital lesions, gonorrhea, chlamydia, CBC, fern test, and nitrazine test.

Preterm labor is considered to be labor commencing after 20 weeks and before 37 weeks gestation. Signs and symptoms of preterm labor should be part of prenatal education commencing at 20 weeks gestation. If there is a single previous preterm labor or birth you should:

- Screen monthly for bacteriuria
- Treat vaginal or cervical infections
- counsel about stress, nutrition, cigarette, alcohol or drug abuse
- reiterate the signs and symptoms of preterm labor

With two or more previous preterm events, or with multiple gestation but no signs of preterm labor, you should also:

- perform a vaginal exam every 2 weeks from 24 weeks gestation onwards to check for cervical changes
- counsel for workload reduction
- recommend condom use
- counsel avoidance of nipple stimulation

### Causes of Preterm Labor

Preterm labor can be caused by a variety of issues. In most cases, however, the cause remains unknown. The following conditions can result in or contribute to preterm labor:

- Vaginal or urinary tract infection progressing into chorioamnionitis and premature rupture of the membranes
- Incompetent cervix
- Polyhydramnios
- Malnutrition and/or dehydration
- Chronic gum disease in the second trimester
- Uterine abnormalities
- Multiple pregnancy
- Improper implantation of the placenta
- Not enough time between pregnancies
- Fetal death
- Extreme or chronic stress, emotional or physical
- Substance abuse

The primary issue is the maturity of the fetal lungs. If development is incomplete, respiratory distress syndrome with retractions, nasal flaring, tachypnea, cyanosis, and grunting on expiration will result.

### Signs and Symptoms of Preterm Labor

A history of the woman's contractions should determine her perception of the duration, frequency, physical location, regularity, and progress to stronger, longer or more frequent. You should then palpate the contractions for intensity, duration and frequency. Perform electronic fetal monitoring and correlate all findings with the palpation results and the woman's perceptions. A very preterm fetus can reposition easily within the uterus and confound monitoring.

Preterm labor is diagnosed when gestation is between 20 and 37 weeks, uterine contractions are 5 to 8 minutes apart or there are four contractions in twenty minutes or eight in sixty minutes, and:

- the membranes are ruptured
- OR membranes are intact and there is progressive cervical change
- OR membranes are intact and the cervix is 2 cm dilated
- OR membranes are intact and there is a positive fFN test.

### Signs Preterm Labor Is Progressing to Birth

Decide the route of birth when fetal presentation and gestational age is determined. Choose analgesia and anesthesia based on the impact to the fetus: do not use narcotics, ataractics, and sedatives prior to delivery. When considering an episiotomy, consider the estimated fetal weight and the condition of the perineum. A pudendal block or local infiltration is recommended unless the mother requires an epidural for comfort and control. In this case, preload the mother with crystalloid IV fluids to alleviate hypotension, although if betamimetics have been administered, consider the increased risk of pulmonary edema. Carefully monitor the fetus which cannot tolerate labor stress like a full term fetus. If a betamimetic drug is used or an intrauterine infection is present, observe for tachycardia. An internal electronic monitor may not be indicated due to skull bone density and structural differences of a preterm fetus.

### *Midwifery Management of Preterm Labor*

Closely conduct your management of preterm labor, and preterm labor that is progressing toward birth with the consulting physician. All treatment decisions work toward a viable infant with the least amount of morbidity. In impending birth, when preterm labor cannot be halted, every decision regarding treatment should avoid fetal asphyxia and trauma.

If there is a history of preterm labor, perform increased monitoring starting at 24 weeks with visits every 2 weeks. Include a gentle cervical exam. Recommend a reduced workload and the use of condoms. If signs of infection appear, screen immediately. If the cervix begins to efface, or if preterm labor is halted, sexual contact should cease and visits become weekly. Give all instructions to the partner and family at each visit. If regular contractions begin or the cervix begins to dilate, immediately contact the consulting physician.

## Tocolytic Therapy

Tocolytic therapy is the administration of certain agents that inhibit uterine contractions. **THESE DRUGS ARE EXTREMELY TOXIC AND MAY PRODUCE DANGEROUS SIDE EFFECTS IN MOTHER AND FETUS.** An early and accurate diagnosis of preterm labor is required. In general, only mothers who are dilated to at least 4 centimeters and are less than 34 weeks gestation are potential candidates for this treatment because it has not been shown to be effective enough to overcome the risk of side effects when used between 34 and 37 weeks, although it may be used under certain conditions. Tocolysis may only prolong pregnancy for 24 to 48 hours, although prolongation of 3 to 7 days has been obtained. When labor has been halted for at least 24 hours corticosteroids can be given which will reduce neonatal mortality, respiratory distress syndrome, and intraventricular hemorrhage in the newborn.

## Tocolytic Agents

Prostaglandin synthesis inhibitors: The most commonly used of these drugs is Indomethacin. They are more effective than other agents at inhibiting uterine contractions. They also have fewer of the severe side effects of betamimetics. These are better choices for women with heart disease, hyperthyroidism, or diabetes but routine use is not encouraged.

Calcium channel blockers: These include nifedipine and nicardepine. There are fewer side effects than betamimetics and magnesium sulfate, and there is little to no adverse effect on fetal outcome. They also postpone birth longer and are as effective as betamimetics and magnesium sulfate in inhibiting uterine contractions and delaying birth making them preferable to betamimetics as tocolytics.

Oxytocin agonists: These are relatively new agents which include atosiban. They appear to have fewer maternal side effects and equal effectiveness in tocolysis but carry greater fetal risk. More extensive study is needed to determine usefulness.

## Beta-Adrenergic Drugs and Magnesium Sulfate

Beta-adrenergic drugs (betamimetics or beta-sympathomimetics): These are the most commonly used drugs and include ritodrine, salbutamol, and terbutaline. Ritodrine has been found to be ineffective and its FDA approval for tocolysis may be reconsidered. These drugs typically have maternal side effects of tachycardia, pulmonary edema, markedly increased cardiac output, blood pressure effects, and increased blood sugar and insulin secretion. Typical fetal side effects are tachycardia, hypoglycemia, and hyperinsulinism after birth. Efforts to maintain pregnancy after stopping preterm labor using beta-adrenergic agonists has proven to be ineffective and is not recommended.

Magnesium sulfate: This has not been evaluated as well as other tocolytic agents and it has some of the most serious side effects including maternal respiratory distress, cardiac arrest and death as well as an increase perinatal morbidity and mortality for the fetus. It is more effectively used for eclampsia.

## Offering Tocolytic Therapy

Prior to tocolytic therapy, it must be decided whether it is best to attempt to stop labor or allow it to continue to birth. The uterine environment must be assessed to determine if it is better for the fetus to remain in utero or if the environment has degenerated to the point where it is better to try to care for the preterm fetus in an intensive care unit with all that this implies to the future development of the baby. Also the side effects and risk of complications to the mother must be kept in mind. Another factor to consider is the time needed to reach an appropriate tertiary care facility or to begin corticosteroid administration for fetal lung maturity issues. If tocolytic therapy is administered, the woman will require increased support, not only due to the emotional issues of preterm labor but also due to physical side effects and complications from the therapy.

## Appropriate Facilities in a Preterm Birth

A level III facility with a neonatal intensive care unit is urgently advised in a preterm birth. Neonatal mortality is significantly reduced when birth takes place at this type of facility as opposed to transporting the newborn there after the birth. Arrangements should be made for a pediatrician or neonatologist to be present at the birth. Consideration for the needs of the neonatal team must be made regarding any delay in clamping and cutting the umbilical cord. A reasonable compromise regarding cord clamping is to hold the baby in a warm blanket below the introitus for 30 to 45 seconds to speed transfusion from the placenta. In case of the need to wait for birth before transporting, arrangements for keeping the baby warm are paramount.

## Hydration and Alcohol Consumption

Hydration is often regarded as a method of stopping preterm labor based on the assumption that preterm labor can begin due to dehydration. However, this has not been shown to be the case, although the recommendation still appears in many texts. Using hydration to attempt to delay birth can increase the risk of pulmonary edema if tocolytic therapy is later used and so can delay the prompt administration of tocolysis when it is needed. The risk of pulmonary edema can be reduced by hydrating intravenously with a hypotonic solution such as 5% dextrose in water or 5% dextrose in 0.25% normal saline.

Prior to the availability of today's tocolytic drugs, alcohol was used to slow or stop preterm labor. It can be given intravenously but oral administration may be effective enough. The equivalent of two shots of strong spirits daily may stall preterm labor.

## Emotional Support in Preterm Labor

You must help the mother allay her fears and anxieties since emotional stress can be a causative agent of preterm labor. An empathetic approach devoid of false reassurances is the best route to take. You can attempt to make the mother feel she has some control over the situation and can positively contribute to its treatment. Trust the mother's suspicions and her reports of any important changes; remain available by phone. If preterm birth does occur, the mother may face separation from the infant although the current trend in "kangaroo care" alleviates this by involving the mother in the care of the infant early and often. The mother may grieve for the loss of the home birth experience and you may be the only person able to listen and give support. At the appropriate time refer the parents to a support organization for parents with premature infants.

### Non-Allopathic Remedies for Preterm Labor

If there is a predisposition towards the condition, consumption of oily fish or fish oil capsules, or supplemental magnesium may help prevent preterm labor. Magnesium supplementation can be used up to 37 weeks gestation; if preterm labor begins, the dosage can be increased and a deep warm bath may help stall labor. Care should be taken with magnesium since it can cause diarrhea. Homeopathic Mag Phos 30C may be effective at a rate of 7 pellets per 4 oz of hot, but not boiling, water. The solution is sipped until gone and the contractions should slow or stop within the hour. Postural tilting several times daily has occasionally stopped preterm labor, perhaps by taking the weight of the fetus off the cervix. If contractions do not slow or if they begin to accelerate notify the consulting physician.

### Bed Rest for Preterm Labor

Studies have shown that placing a mother on prolonged bed rest does not prevent preterm labor. It may, in fact, be deleterious because the lack of activity can decrease the muscle strength required for birth and postpartum. It can also increase the risk of clots in the veins of the legs. However, if a mother presents with signs and symptoms of preterm labor, bed rest should be prescribed until it is determined whether the criteria for preterm labor has been met. The mother should be placed in the lateral, or side-lying, position with external FHT and uterine contractility monitoring. If the membranes are still intact, vaginal exams to monitor for cervical changes may be performed, preferably by the same examiner each time.

### Postdate Pregnancy

A postdate pregnancy is one which has surpassed 42 weeks. There may be a family history of postdate infants, no reason and no abnormal findings, or the mother may not yet be ready for the pregnancy to end. While the fetus may continue to grow, the risk of cephalopelvic disproportion or shoulder dystocia increases. The mother may decrease her fluid and food intake in an effort to keep the fetal size down and risk fetal weight loss, cord compression from oligohydramnios, fetal distress or stillbirth (all included in fetal postmaturity syndrome). If there are no mitigating factors other than postdatism, practice watchful waiting. Assessments to monitor fetal health include fetal kick-counts, a non-stress test, and serial ultrasounds to check amniotic fluid volume. If no abnormality is found, home-based induction can be attempted, especially if the fetus is becoming large or if the head is well into the pelvis. Or waiting can be continued.

### Postdate Pregnancy

A postdate pregnancy is one that has surpassed 294 days beyond the last accurately dated menstrual period or 280 days beyond the date of ovulation or fertilization. There are several terms for a postdate pregnancy: prolonged pregnancy, postterm pregnancy, and postmaturity. It is important to recognize that postdate pregnancy and postmaturity syndrome are two separate conditions. Postdate pregnancy, even when called postmaturity, is a prenatal condition whereas postmaturity syndrome is a condition diagnosed in the infant upon neonatal examination. The percentage of postdate pregnancies is 1% to 3% when the pregnancy is accurately dated and the menstrual and ultrasound findings are consistent. In addition, the optimal range of gestational ages for human gestation is not known. The definition of postdates as pregnancies that persist 2 weeks past the estimated date of birth without labor is arbitrary.

## Labor Induction in a Postdate Pregnancy

In most cases, it is best to allow labor to begin spontaneously as long as there are no complications arising. However, in some cases, there is justification for inducing labor. The following issues may indicate a need to induce labor:

- A low biophysical profile score which translates into a nonreassuring test result for the fetus
- Preeclampsia that progressively worsens at term
- Oligohydramnios
- Insulin dependent diabetes
- History of previous stillbirth at term
- Intrauterine growth restriction

It may also be justified in the case of a woman with a history of rapid labor who has an effaced cervix at 4 cm dilation who may go into labor away from medical assistance. Being tired of pregnancy and the attendant discomfort or feeling as though waiting is causing family difficulty is not a justification for induction, but rather a need for more support.

## Risks of True Postdate Pregnancy

An increased risk of stillbirth has been found in postdate pregnancy which may be attributed to uteroplacental insufficiency. This eventually causes fetal hypoxia. In addition, amniotic fluid levels drop significantly in the final few weeks of gestation, increasing the risk of cord compression, especially during labor, as well as the risk of meconium aspiration pneumonia from inhalation of a viscous meconium stained fluid that is less dilute than usual owing to low fluid levels. In some postdate neonates there is a loss of subcutaneous fat as in postmaturity syndrome while others suffer macrosomia which can lead to cephalopelvic disproportion or shoulder dystocia. In many instances the true risk is during labor when the stresses to the fetus are significant and exacerbate any fetal compromise.

## Active Management of a Postdate Pregnancy

Once the 42$^{nd}$ week of gestation has been reached with no labor commencing, active management of the pregnancy can be justified. If the cervix is ripe, the mother may try self-inducing labor by ingesting castor oil to stimulate the onset as early as 40 weeks as long as you both concur with this treatment. At 41 weeks or beyond, you may strip the membranes. If the cervix is not ripe, prostaglandin gel or inserts, such as Cervadil, may be implanted into the birth canal anticipating induction of labor at 41 to 42 weeks. If you, the mother, and the consulting physician concur, pitocin induction may be scheduled when 42 weeks is reached without spontaneous labor. If dates are accurate, the pregnancy should not be allowed to go beyond 42 complete weeks.

## Anticipatory Management of the Postdate Pregnancy

When the pregnancy continues to be normal with no indications that induction should occur, there are several assessments that should be made on a regular basis once the 40$^{th}$ week of gestation has been reached with no sign of labor. To reassure the mother, the true measure of the estimated date of birth should be reviewed to establish understanding that the estimation encompasses a range of time, not a single date. Review the postdate management plan with her and document her acceptance of the plan. Perform nonstress tests and measurements of amniotic fluid volume twice weekly starting at the 41$^{st}$ week and continuing until birth. Perform a full biophysical profile and contact the consulting physician if the nonstress test or amniotic fluid volume is not reassuring. If labor has not begun by 42 weeks and the dating of the pregnancy is accurate, notify the consulting physician and being active management of the pregnancy.

## Non-Hormonal Methods of Stimulating Labor

These are non-hormonal alternatives to labor induction.

- Nipple stimulation: Several methods have been recommended for stimulating the nipples, from using a breast pump to various types of breast massage. Caution should be used to avoid hyperstimulation of the uterus.
- Castor oil: ingestion of 60 mg of castor oil in apple or orange juice has been shown to stimulate spontaneous labor in term pregnancy. Onset of action is 2 to 6 hours. There appear to be few complications to this method.
- Foley bulb or balloon catheter: The catheter is used as a mechanical device to stretch the cervix. The advantages are the ease and safety of use, the lack of expense, and the ease of placement and removal. Fetal monitoring is not required.
- Sexual stimulation: When the pregnancy is uncomplicated and the membranes are intact, there is no contraindication to sexual manipulation or stimulation in an effort to induce labor.
- Membrane stripping: a method of separating the membranes from the bottom of the cervix in order to achieve a physical prostaglandin release to trigger labor. It may reduce gestation by 2 to 5 days. It should not be done if premature membrane rupture will endanger the mother or fetus, if cervicitis is present, if there is a low lying placenta or placenta previa, undiagnosed vaginal bleeding, or unknown lie of the fetus.
- Amniotomy: artificial rupture of membranes (AROM). The membranes are ruptured in an attempt to stimulate labor. The risks are the same as premature rupture of the membranes. This procedure is contraindicated in a non-vertex lie, an unengaged head, or small fetus due to risk of cord prolapse. Better outcomes are associated with AROM at 5 cm or larger cervical dilation. It is not recommended as a sole method of induction.

## Hormonal Methods of Labor Induction

Vaginal delivery is more likely to occur if the cervix is softened, or "ripe". The Bishop scoring system assigns a point value to the centimeters of dilation, the percentage of effacement, the station, the cervical consistency, and the fetal position. Thirteen is the maximum possible score. A common Bishop score for beginning oxytocin administration is six (6). Cervadil and Prepidil, both PGE2 compounds for cervical ripening, are used to prepare an unripe cervix prior to labor induction. This increases the likelihood of a vaginal delivery when labor is induced. Most hormonal methods of labor induction are more stressful than natural or spontaneous labor. The rate of analgesia increases in these cases. Oxytocin is the most common medication used for labor induction. Also known as Pitocin, oxytocin is administered in various protocols according to facility or physician preference. You should be cognizant of the protocols in use in your community.

## Non-Allopathic Methods of Inducing Labor

Evening primrose oil, taken internally, has long been a recommended herbal method of ripening the uterus which may lead to spontaneous labor. This method may take up to a week to soften the cervix. This same herbal oil may be massaged into the cervix to help it to soften in preparation for dilation. Black cohosh tincture is stronger and may product results within 3 or 4 hours. Blue cohosh tincture has also been used to induce labor as has homeopathic Caulophyllum, 30C or 200x, or Cimicifuga 30C. Acupuncture, blue cohosh enemas, abdominal massage, and visualizing the uterus contracting have all been used to induce labor without external hormonal stimulation or other intervention. There is little evidence that physical activity appropriate for a woman at term will initiate labor.

## Osteopathy, Chiropractic and Reflexology Treatment

Midwives typically do not practice osteopathy or chiropractic but may make a referral to a practitioner. Both practices rebalance the neuromusculoskeletal system to align the body. The difference is osteopathy looks at mobility in joints where chiropractic treats the relative position of joints. While both practices have been used to treat symptoms of heartburn, nausea and constipation, they more often deal with structural symptoms such as backaches and sciatica. These practices can also be used in labor. Some osteopaths specialize in craniosacral therapy which treats infants with excessive head molding after instrument deliveries.

Reflexology uses very precise manipulation of the feet to treat general physiological discomfort and labor pain. Constipation, headaches, anxiety, sciatica and migraines are eased using reflexology. Some research has shown an easier labor for women regularly treated with reflexology than in the average population. There are some contraindications and possible complications if used inappropriately.

## Acupuncture in Pregnancy and Childbirth

Acupuncture is based on the principle of meridians, or energy lines, running through organs in the body. Stress causes obstructions on a meridian. If the point of the obstruction can be stimulated, by a needle or acupressure, the energies will be rebalanced. Other methods of stimulation are using suction cups to cover the point or by applying heat through the use of moxa sticks. Acupuncture has been used to relieve pregnancy related nausea by using acupressure on a point on the wrist. For a more complete use of this treatment, a qualified traditional acupuncturist should be consulted.

Acupuncture used in labor has been useful for pain relief, labor induction and acceleration of labor, as well as treatment for a retained placenta. Pain relief can take effect as quickly as 40 minutes and last as much as 6 hours with no drugs.

## Tubal Pregnancy

A ruptured tube is life threatening to the mother.  The fetus will be lost and the mother may suffer severe internal hemorrhage leading to shock and/or death. When notified of symptoms indicative of tubal pregnancy or rupture, call the consulting physician immediately and instruct the mother to call an ambulance. Under no circumstances is she or anyone else to drive to the emergency room. If the tube has not ruptured, the embryo will be surgically removed or methotrexate will be administered to dissolve the embryo. Refer the mother, her partner, and her family for support and counseling following this incident to help with the impact of nearly dying, losing a baby, and possibly losing her fertility. In recent years, ultrasound imaging has assisted in diagnosing tubal pregnancies earlier and alleviating the worst of the outcomes.

### *Characteristics and Symptoms of Tubal Pregnancy*

A tubal pregnancy is a form of ectopic pregnancy in which the embryo develops in the Fallopian tube. Bimanual exam shows a luteal mass. Tubal pregnancies account for up to 95% of all ectopic pregnancies. As the embryo grows, it may be expelled into the abdominal cavity or the tube will rupture when the embryo grows too large, around 10 to 13 weeks gestation. Tubal pregnancy symptoms:

- pelvic pain
- shoulder pain
- spot bleeding
- high degree of shock after rupture, differentiating it from abortion

Pelvic inflammatory disease is a major cause of tubal pregnancy. Scar tissue may partially obstruct some areas of the tubes leaving blind pockets or reduced numbers of cilia.

Other causes are:

- STD infections
- trauma from IUDs
- infection after abortion
- progesterone based birth control
- reconstructive surgery from a prior tube rupture
- DES exposure
- assisted reproduction

Conditions that mimic tubal pregnancy symptoms are pelvic inflammatory disease, appendicitis, and severe gastrointestinal illness.

## Hydatidiform Mole

A hydatidiform mole is created by abnormal development of the chorionic villi which then fills the uterus with clear, spherical vesicles. The most common presentation is a complete mole; there is no fetus, instead the mole forms due to inactivation of the chromosomes of the ovum by an abnormal sperm. This occurs in 95% of all molar pregnancies. In the remaining 5%, a partial mole develops with some fetal tissue containing abnormal numbers of chromosomes. The fetus rarely survives.

Molar pregnancy symptoms include:

- Light brown bleeding that may last for weeks.
- The uterus is unusually large for dates and feels woody or doughy to the touch.
- Abnormally high hCG levels caused by the abnormal chorionic villi growth.
- Hypertension and proteinuria due to liver stress.
- Hyperemesis occurs in 25-35% of cases.

Molar pregnancies usually spontaneously abort but surgical removal may be required. Molar pregnancies can develop into invasive cancer 20% of the time.

## Ectopic Pregnancy

An ectopic pregnancy is one that occurs outside of the uterus. In 95% of cases the pregnancy occurs in the Fallopian tube (tubal pregnancy). Alternatively, the embryo may implant in the ovary, cervix, or abdomen. It is estimated that ectopic pregnancies occur in 1.5% of all pregnancies. Early diagnosis and treatment is crucial to avoid extreme maternal morbidity and mortality. Any unexplained abdominal pain and bleeding early in the pregnancy should alert you to the possibility of an ectopic pregnancy. Additional symptoms include gastrointestinal upset, vomiting, and diarrhea.

Cervical pregnancy and abdominal pregnancy, both very rare, can cause massive hemorrhage. Abdominal pregnancy can also result in infection followed by peritonitis and septicemia.

Extremely rarely, the fetus goes to term but with intrauterine growth restriction deformities due to lack of an amniotic fluid sac. Delivery is by laparotomy. The placenta may be left in place to degenerate since removal can elicit uncontrollable hemorrhage.

### Placental Abruption

Placental abruption is the separation of a normally implanted placenta after the 22nd week of gestation. Preeclampsia, sudden decrease in uterine size, and trauma are often implicated. A previous caesarian section can increase the risk of placental abruption by 40%. Cigarette smoking may also be a factor. Bleeding from a partial separation can increase the separation when pressure from the hemorrhage pushes the placenta away from the uterine wall. Blood may drain through the vagina or infiltrate into the myometrium causing hypovolemic shock.

Placental abruption is classified in two ways. The first is classification by type of blood loss: revealed, concealed, or mixed hemorrhage. Blood loss occurring vaginally is visible and classified as revealed. Concealed blood loss occurs when the blood is entrapped. A mixed hemorrhage is one where blood loss is both revealed and concealed. Another classification is by degree of separation: mild, moderate, and severe. The most severe type of hemorrhage is concealed.

### Types of Placental Abruption

In mild placental abruption the mother and fetus are stable with no maternal shock or fetal compromise; the uterus feels normal and there is no abdominal pain. Bleeding occurs: perform constant fetal monitoring. If gestation is less than 37 weeks a hospital stay may be needed and the mother allowed to go home if bleeding ceases. If gestation is at or beyond 37 weeks, induction may be offered. Heavy bleeding or fetal distress may dictate a caesarian section.

Moderate abruption often means significant blood loss, fetal hypoxia or demise, maternal shock, and abdominal tenderness. Address all issues. A caesarian section may be required if the fetus is alive and the mother stable. If the fetus is in either very good condition or dead, a vaginal delivery may be advantageous.

### Assessment in Placental Abruption

Fetal movement may become excessive then cease due to hypoxia. Failure to elicit fetal heart tones with a stethoscope, fetoscope or dopplar is not necessarily a sign of fetal demise. Electronic fetal monitoring and ultrasound to assess the fetal heart can give more complete information about fetal well-being and mortality. If fetal death has occurred, do not attempt to hide this information from the mother for any reason or length of time.

There may be maternal history or symptoms of preeclampsia, headaches, nausea, and vomiting. There may be trauma due to accidents or domestic violence. External cephalic version, birth of a first twin, and loss of large volumes of amniotic fluid can cause placental abruption. Maternal shock may occur. Previously high blood pressure may now be in normal range. The uterus may be enlarged with a concealed hemorrhage; it may be hard and guarded. Minimize palpation to avoid further trauma. Severe hemorrhage commonly leads to fetal death.

### Placenta Previa

Placenta previa is a condition in which the placenta implants in the lower section of the uterus and partially or completely covers the cervical os. The uterine wall stretches and grows during pregnancy. The placenta will shift position with it and may separate and hemorrhage in the third trimester. Placenta previa is more common with:

- maternal age over 35
- multiparity
- history of placenta previa
- multiple gestation

- smoking
- previous uterine surgery

Bleeding is sudden and painless. There is often fetal malpresentation. Ultrasound can diagnose placenta previa early in the pregnancy which must be confirmed later in pregnancy. If it still covers the os vaginal birth is contraindicated. When painless third trimester bleeding is reported, a vaginal exam should not be performed until placental position is confirmed. If placenta previa is ruled out you may perform a digital exam.

If placenta previa is diagnosed in the third trimester and the cervical os remains covered, vaginal birth is contraindicated. If the placenta moves away from the os and no other symptoms, such as bleeding, occur, vaginal birth may be attempted with careful observation for cord presentation or other cord issue. If bleeding is reported management should consider gestational age, severity of bleeding, and fetal status. At 37 weeks or more, a caesarian section is advised. If bleeding resolves prior to birth, the fetus must be monitored closely. If fetal distress does not resolve, delivery must occur. If bleeding stops and the uterus does not begin to contract, home bed-rest may be permitted as long as 24 hour access to emergency transport is available. In some cases hospitalization until gestational maturity will be required along with pelvic rest.

## PROM

While premature rupture of the membranes is technically defined as the rupture of the membranes prior to the onset of labor, in practice it is often defined in consideration of the number of hours between rupture and labor onset. The period in between is called the latent period and typically lasts from 1 to 12 hours or more. If the pregnancy is not yet term, the condition may be called preterm premature rupture of the membranes (PPROM). If the membranes rupture more than 24 hours prior to the commencement of labor, the condition is called prolonged rupture of the membranes. There is increased risk of PROM with incompetent cervix, fetal malpresentation, vaginal/cervical infection, polyhydramios, and multiple gestation. Nulliparous women are at greater risk of preterm premature rupture of the membranes due to occupational fatigue. This does not affect multiparous women.

### *Management Options*

PROM becomes more difficult to diagnose unless leaking fluid is visible in the os 6 to 12 hours after the rupture. Rupture is diagnostic of premature rupture of the membranes in and of itself. If fluid is not visible, a positive fern test and a history with likely conditions will suffice. Chorioamnionitis risk is increased with each vaginal exam, so minimize them. If the latent period lasts beyond 72 hours, fetal mortality increases significantly. Management takes into consideration the differences in infection rates with PROM before and after 37 weeks gestation and its latent period. Management options include:

- Ensuring birth within 24 hours of rupture
- Awaiting spontaneous labor while monitoring for signs of chorioamnionitis

A digital exam for cervical dilation is unnecessary unless induction is chosen. Perform the exam at the time of induction in this case. Ultrasound can confirm presentation. If the FTH is abnormal, a digital exam is warranted to check for cord prolapse.

### *Identification*

Premature rupture of the membranes increases the risk of infection. Diagnosis includes:

- A history including the amount of lost fluid, inability to control the leakage with Kegel exercises (differentiates from urine flow), time of the rupture, the color (clear, cloudy, yellow or green) and odor of the fluid (musty), and time of last sexual intercourse (differentiates from semen).
- Abdominal palpation to determine fluid volume. Differentiates a frank rupture from a leak.
- A sterile speculum exam to check the external genitalia, cervical os, and vaginal vault for fluid, to observe any fluid expulsion under pressure, to observe any fluid for vernix or lanugo if gestational age is more than 32 weeks, to check for cervical dilation, prolapsed cord or presenting fetal parts.
- Acquisition of samples and images such as a fern test, nitrazine paper test, an ultrasound for oligohydramnios, and specimens for Group B Streptococcus.

### *Non-Allopathic Treatment*

The greatest threat after rupture is fetal and maternal sepsis. Caution the mother to:

- avoid tub baths until advanced labor
- use increased vigilance in hygiene when using the bathroom, using sterilized toilet paper if desired (toilet paper that has been baked at 200 degrees for 1 hour)
- avoid hand-to-genitalia contact, underwear, and pads unless flowing heavily, then the pad should be changed frequently
- remain hydrated
- increase vitamin C consumption to 250 mg every 24 hours
- eat non-constipating foods
- monitor her temperature every 3 to 4 hours

A daily CBC may be required. After 24 hours have passed since rupture, check the FHT regularly. Other alternative therapies include supplemental vitamin E along with the vitamin C, ingesting 5 to 10 drops of Echinacea tincture 2 to 3 times a day to prevent infection, and drinking Nettle, Comfrey, or Violet leaf infusions for healing.

## Incompetent Cervical Os

An incompetent cervical os (incompetent cervix) is diagnosed when the cervix effaces and dilates in the second or early third trimester without pain. The symptoms often include vaginal bleeding, ruptured membranes, or pelvic pressure. Risk factors include a history of abortion at 14 or more weeks of gestation or cervical laceration after a vaginal or caesarian birth, extreme distension of the cervix during a prolonged second stage labor in a previous pregnancy, multiple elective abortions in the first or second trimester, exposure to DES, or extreme cervical conization. If the membranes are still intact and the cervix is in an appropriate condition, an incompetent cervix is often treated with cervical cerclage sometimes called a purse-string.

## Cephalopelvic Disproportion, Cerclage, and DIC

Cephalopelvic disproportion is a disparity between the size of the mother's pelvis and the size of the fetal head.

Cerclage is a non-absorbable suture inserted into the cervix to keep it closed in the case of incompetent cervix. Incompetent cervix may be caused by cone biopsy, trauma during a D&C or induced abortion. It can also be a congenital weakness of the cervix.

Disseminated Intravascular Coagulation (DIC): If abnormal blood clotting occurs in the blood vessels, the coagulation cascade is disrupted, clotting factors are used up and the blood loses the ability to clot, thereby causing severe hemorrhage. In pregnancy, this can occur if a miscarriage or stillbirth occurs and all products of conception are not expelled from the uterus within 3 to 4 weeks of the fetal death.

## Management of PROM Once Labor Commences

Once labor commences after premature rupture of the membranes management is normal with the following exceptions:

- Assess temperature and pulse every 2 hours
- Monitor FHR every hour prior to onset of labor. For induction, the FHR is monitored more closely, even constantly with electronic monitoring
- Avoid vaginal exams if possible
- If a vaginal exam is performed observe the temperature of the vaginal walls, and the odor and color of the discharge or fluid
- Monitor hydration levels closely

If gestation is at least 36 weeks with no other complications, and the mother has chosen spontaneous labor, she may go home to wait while monitoring for infection. A hospital stay is required with infection. FHT is checked every 4 hours and maternal testing follows local practice. If gestation is less than 36 weeks, the pregnancy is prolonged while watching for infection. Notify the consulting physician if the premature rupture is preterm or prolonged.

## Emergency Situations Requiring Immediate Call

These are emergencies. Parents should be instructed to call the midwife at once if they observe:

- Vaginal bleeding indicating possible miscarriage, spontaneous abortion, or a molar or ectopic pregnancy. In later trimesters, placenta previa, placental abruption, or a ruptured cervical polyp may be indicated.
- Blisters breaking out in the perineal or anal area indicating herpesvirus.
- Severe pelvic or abdominal pain indicating a tubal pregnancy or placental abruption depending on the trimester.
- Persistent, severe pain in the mid-back indicating pyelonephritis or kidney infection.
- Swollen hands and face, severe headaches, blurry vision, or pain under the ribcage indicating pre-eclampsia.
- A gush of fluid in the first or second trimester indicating a miscarriage.
- Premature delivery in the late second or early third trimester indicating a miscarriage.
- Regular uterine contractions before 37 weeks indicating impending premature birth.
- Cessation of fetal movement indicating fetal demise.

# Labor, Birth and Immediate Postpartum

## Hydrotherapy and Visualization During Labor

Hydrotherapy, or immersion in water, can relieve muscle spasms and the effects of gravity on the woman's body decreasing the stress on the pelvis. There is little evidence in the literature of increased risk with hydrotherapy. The use of warm water to soothe tight muscles and uncomfortable joints can decrease reliance on analgesics. Labor progresses more efficiently and quickly when the mother is relaxed, thereby negating use of labor augmentation drugs. The mother's birth experience is also more positive. The temperature of the water should not be above normal body temperature. This avoids increasing fetal temperature and heart rate. Continuous soaking can slow labor somewhat so the length of the bath should be monitored and bathing delayed until labor is well established.

Visualization is the practice of visualizing a soothing place or a smooth birth. It is often taught in conjunction with muscle relaxation techniques to help the mother achieve a positive birth experience.

## General and OB Backrub

The general backrub is a simple, overall backrub intended to promote relaxation. The "OB" backrub is a method of applying pressure to specific areas of the lower spine as advised by the mother. The fetal head generates pressure against the spine causing a localized pain that can be pinpointed and communicated by the mother. The mother should also be in control of the amount of pressure required to counter the pressure of the fetal head without causing additional discomfort. Typically the OB rub is only needed during contractions. If the woman is supine, a small folded towel or tennis balls can be placed under the area where there is pressure.

## Tub Bath During Active Labor

Once active labor has begun, there is no reason an ambulatory mother cannot relax in a tub of warm water. This is a very relaxing comfort measure. The water must be deep enough to cover the abdomen creating a buoyancy and hydrotherapeutic lift to relieve pressure. A Jacuzzi or tub designed for labor and birth are excellent ways to provide this if available. Relaxation can help the cervix dilate more rapidly and effectively. However, after about 2 hours, contractions may begin to stall. At that time the mother should leave the tub to stimulate further labor. If the birth partner wishes to be involved and has not yet found a way, sharing the bath can be an intimate and supportive activity.

## Communication in the Birth Environment

Whenever speaking to the mother during labor, kind and encouraging words in a firm easily heard voice are the most helpful. Particularly for the first time mother, this is a time when she may feel out of control or, even if well educated about the birth process, unprepared for the sensations of labor. She may lack the confidence to apply what she has learned at the appropriate time. With calm encouragement, she can find her way in this new realm. Sometimes the best communication is silence. The mother may feel overwhelmed by the smallest suggestion, or, if there have been many visitors or much chaos, she may welcome the lack of sound to help her focus on her labor. Music can be a way of relaxing whenever a time of rest is available, especially if the music is meaningful to the mother.

## Mobility During Labor

Many studies have shown that mobility during labor enhances the birth experience and the outcome. Women who are allowed to remain ambulatory when desired during labor experienced:

- Fewer caesarian sections and episiotomies
- Less need for labor augmentation or induction
- Shorter labors
- Less need for analgesia
- Fewer issues with fetal compromise
- More effective uterine action

The upright position during labor alleviates problems with supine hypotension, reduced pelvic outlet space, perineal trauma, and less effective uterine contractions. The upright position takes advantage of both gravity to help engage the fetal head and the movement of walking to distribute the pressure of the head across the cervix to allow for coordinate and effective uterine contractions.

There may be contraindications to ambulation. These should be considered on an individual basis according to the physical condition of the mother and fetus.

## Abdominal Breathing and Panting

Abdominal breathing can be taught to any mother with no prenatal breathing training. Abdominal breathing has two modes of action: performing controlled breathing will serve as a distraction from the pain of contractions and it helps lift the diaphragm off the uterus to relieve pressure and pain. Once transition is reached, however, the mother cannot continue abdominal breathing. At this point, some form of panting is required, either the pant-pant-blow rhythm, if possible, or panting "like a dog", whichever the mother is capable of. Panting is for those times when the mother is asked not to push. This includes when the cervix has not yet fully dilated, during delivery of the head between contractions, and if the cord is around the baby's neck and must be clamped and cut prior to delivery of the body. The best teaching method is to demonstrate and breath with the mother at each contraction.

## Non-Allopathic Treatment for Pain Relief

Homeopathic Arnica 200C alleviates irritation and reduces swelling in the cervix making contractions more effective and regular. Motherwort tincture provides pain relief when birth is not imminent and rest is needed. It creates a somewhat disconnected feeling to the uterus however, and may be contraindicated if labor is not yet regular. Skullcap tincture is a good overall pain reliever but has a sedative effect. Back, side, and uterine spasms may respond to a tincture of St. Joan's Wort which works well in combination with Skullcap.

Other pain relief measures include acupuncture, reflexology, and aromatherapy. All should be given by trained personnel. Full body acupuncture is often used but ear lobe acupuncture may be sufficient and is easily learned. Aromatherapy uses essential oils for massage, in baths, or applied to mucus membranes. Reflexology, which involves pressure or massage on very specific areas of the feet, has been found to alleviate some pain issues in labor.

## Maternal Positioning During Labor

Allow the mother to assume the position she wishes if possible. It is likely that she will instinctively seek the position most suitable for her at a given point in labor. You can still offer support by suggesting positions that will alleviate pressure due to various fetal positions. Possibilities include supine with any or no incline, knee-chest, all-fours, lateral recumbent, sitting, standing, walking or squatting. Rotation of the fetus to an anterior position may be accomplished by the mother leaning forward, supported by a partner, table, birthing ball, or other support. The hands-and-knees or knees-chest position may also accomplish this. Lateral recumbent positions can help rotate a fetus from an occipital posterior position. Once transition has occurred and second stage labor commences, you should be ready to assist with delivery from any position the mother may take be it hands-knees, squatting or any other position the mother feels is best.

## Herbal and Homeopathic Support for Labor

For intense early labor, Cimicifuga 200C reduces intensity and establishes an effective rhythm. Caulophyllum 200C encourages regular contractions. Pulsatilla 200C helps inconsistent early labor and emotional tensions.

For active labor, Sepia 200C reduces the mother's fears of the intensity of contractions. If birth seems imminent, Gelsimium 200C administration facilitates cervical dilation and effacement. If dilation is incomplete but the mother desires pushing, Arnica 200C will prevent cervical swelling. If there is a strong urge to push at 6 or 7 cm dilation, Sepia and Arnica administered together with repeated administration of Sepia every 10 to 15 minutes reduces swelling and inhibits tension. Treat exhaustion with China, Carbo Veg, or Ustilago plus an enema of warm water and honey, or some royal jelly taken orally. Essence of Chicken may also help.

Caulophyllum can help labor continue and reduce the risk of postpartum hemorrhage. Aconite calms the mother. Arnica helps with pain, uneven contractions, and swelling.

## First Stage Labor

First stage labor may last hours and the mother may need reminding that she will require rest and nutrition to maintain her energy for later stages of labor and birthing. She should be encouraged to sleep if laboring at night and rest between contractions during the day. As labor progresses, the mother will choose positions to labor in that seem right to her but if nonproductive positions are taken up too often, she may need encouragement to shift to a better position to help labor continue effectively. If labor seems to have stalled, physical activity, such as walking, can help stimulate labor and give the mother a change of scenery.

## Physical Assessments Required in Early Labor

Notes should be taken regarding how labor started and its progress. Between contractions:

- the mother's urine should be checked for ketones
- her blood pressure, pulse and temperature taken
- the baby should be palpated for position and descent

During and immediately after contractions, fetal heart tones should be taken to assess fetal response. The uterus may also be palpated to gauge the intensity of the contraction. Vaginal exams should be done sparingly at this time of labor and should have maternal consent. The exam should start as a contraction ends. The dilation should be gauged in centimeters, and the quality and placement of the cervical os should be noted. Most importantly, estimates should be taken of effacement, station of the head, and how evenly the head fills the pelvic cavity. Findings should be interpreted depending on the rapidity of labor and the mother's response to the labor.

### Frequency of Vital Signs During First Stage Labor

Maternal blood pressure is usually checked every hour, while the temperature, pulse and respirations are checked every 2 to 4 hours if the temperature is normal and the membranes are intact.

Once the membranes have ruptured, temperature, pulse, and respirations are checked every 1 to 2 hours. Each time the mother passes urine during labor, it should be tested by dipstick for ketones indicating exhaustion or distress and proteins indicating preeclampsia. The labor record should also be updated with fluid intake, urinary output, and any emesis in general so that dehydration and ketosis can be avoided.

### Membranes and Uterine Contraction

The membranes typically rupture by the end of the first stage of labor. If the membranes rupture prior to the onset of labor it is termed premature rupture of the membranes (PROM); in 80% of PROM cases, labor begins spontaneously within 24 hours.

Early contractions are irregular with short duration, every 20 to 30 minutes and lasting 15 to 20 seconds with mild intensity. By the end of the first stage of labor, the contractions are regular with longer duration and intensity, every 2 to 3 minutes and lasting 60 to 90 seconds with severe intensity. There are variations in this pattern from woman to woman. The normal uterine contraction pattern, called the normal gradient pattern, develops synchronous activity in which the contraction is longer and harder at the top of the fundus and gradually decreases in duration and intensity through the midportion until it ceases towards the cervix.

### Fetal Heart Tones During First Stage Labor

Fetal well-being should be checked whenever a vaginal exam is performed during labor. The fetal heart tones should be evaluated using a fetoscope or Dopplar every 30 minutes during active labor. Unless there are indications of complications continuous electronic fetal monitoring is not required and in fact, can create a situation where the mother is not able to move as she needs. Additional observations should be taken when the membranes rupture, whenever there is a sudden change in labor patterns or contractions, whenever maternal medication is administered and at its peak, after enema expulsion, and any time there is an obstetric or medical complication beginning.

### Fetal Lie, Presentation, Position and Descent

The normal fetal lie is longitudinal with vertex cephalic presentation, accounting for about 95% of all longitudinal lies. About 66% will be positioned with the occiput in the left of the mother's pelvis with the rest positioned in the right. The most common position at the commencement of labor is left occiput transverse (LOT) because the head typically enters the pelvic inlet with the occiput to the transverse portion of the mother's pelvis. Breech presentation at the start of labor accounts for about 3 to 3.5 % of mothers. One half percent are face presentations. The majority of the remaining is typically transverse and oblique lies which are abnormal in labor and require referral to the consulting physician. Generally, the outcome is caesarian section. Vaginal examination after the cervix has started to dilate will confirm definitive diagnoses of the presentation, position, and variety determined during abdominal palpation.

### Vasa Previa Presentation

In vasa previa presentations, the placental or cord vessels present over the cervical os. It is a very rare occurrence that can happen with a velamentous cord insertion or if the vessels emerge beyond the edge of the placenta, running through membranes immediately above the cervix to an accessory succenturiate lob of placental tissue. This condition may be diagnosed if a pulse is felt near the cervix prior to labor or may remain undetected until early labor. If the membrane ruptures near where the vessels run, the mother can hemorrhage and the baby will die. If bleeding is noted after membrane rupture, the mother should be administered oxygen and transported to the hospital. The backup physician must be consulted anytime a presenting part cannot be identified or that may be abnormal.

### Compound Presentation

Compound presentation means that a hand (most usually) presents alongside the head in the birth canal. This is called a "nuchal hand" or "nuchal arm". This is usually not diagnosed until the head is birthing depending on how far down the hand is. If the head and arm are not yet engaged, the Scott and Sutton's hip-twist movement may suffice to correct this presentation. Because the arm in addition to the head creates such a large circumference perineal tearing is more likely. If the hip-twist does not resolve the issue, the baby's fingers should be pinched in an attempt to cause the hand to retract. If it does not, the arm should be extracted so the shoulders can be born.

### Face Presentation

In face presentation, the deflexed head is evident during prenatal palpation unless the baby is posterior. If it is discovered before the head is fixed into the pelvis, an attempt should be made to secure flexion. Face presentation can be caused by inlet CPD (cephalopelvic distortion) or a cord around the neck which will tighten and deflex the head as it descends. Fetal heart tones must be monitored closely and the birth should not be rushed. Face presentation occurs in 4% of births and can cause a serious obstruction requiring transport to a hospital prior to delivery. The baby must be born chin up to prevent the brow from becoming lodged in the symphysis. This presentation causes extra strain on the perineum and tearing may be unavoidable. The baby will receive more fluids than usual into the nose during birth, requiring more suction and possibly resuscitation. The bruising and swelling can be treated with arnica and Vitamin K.

### Effacement and Dilation of the Cervix

Effacement and dilation are the result of uterine contractions and progressive effacement and dilation are the only indications of true labor. It is assessed in percentages: no effacement is "0% effaced", complete effacement is "100% effaced".

Dilation is caused by uterine contractions and the pressure of the membranes, or the presenting part if the membranes are ruptured, on the cervical os. Dilation is assessed by measuring the diameter of the cervix in centimeters. 0 cm is closed, 10 cm is complete dilation. A primagravida often presents 50 to 60% effaced and up to 1 cm dilation prior to labor due to Braxton Hicks. Progression is sequential then sudden with 50 to 100% effacement occurring, then dilation completing. A multigravida may present with no effacement and 1-2 cm dilation when entering labor.

### Visual Technique of Estimating Dilation

In order to avoid internal exams during labor, a visual technique can be used to estimate dilation. It is based on observation of the area directly above the mother's anus. A dilation progresses, a dark red line will be seen to extend up towards and between the buttocks. When it reaches the sacrococcygeal joint, dilation is complete. This technique supports the forward leaning positions and has been found to be reliable. A second visual cue can be observed if the mother is upright; a crease will develop just above and parallel to the pubic bone, extending completely across the lower abdomen when dilation is complete. The fetus is likely passing through the spines if the head is no longer palpable above the pubic bone or if the shoulders seem to be rotating upon palpation.

## STATION OF THE PRESENTING PART

The station of the presenting part is measured in centimeters from above or below the ischial spines. The ischial spines represent 0 station. Above the spines is station -1 through -5, below the spine is station +1 through +5. -5 is an unengaged floating presenting part whereas +5 is the presenting part at the vaginal orifice. Engagement is the point where the widest portion of the presenting part has passed through the pelvic inlet, not the point where the presenting part is at station 0. If there is significant fetal skull molding and caput succedaneum, the station may be difficult to determine.

## HOMEOPATHIC TREATMENT FOR DEHYDRATION AND VOMITING

Homeopathic China, Carbo Veg, or Ustilago 200C will alleviate dehydration and exhaustion. It has been found that ice chips actually intensify the desire for liquids rather than relieving thirst and dehydration. Sips of water or other clear liquid with some sugar added for energy are better treatments for dehydration, dry mouth and throat, although unrestricted access to liquids would be best if possible.

Herbs that have often been used to alleviate nausea and vomiting are peppermint, spearmint, or chamomile tea, and ginger capsules or tea. Nausea can also be relieved by pressure on the acupressure point PC-6 on the inner wrist. Nausea may be due to an empty stomach. Food restrictions may not be necessary in the first stage of labor. Light, non-constipating foods help supply energy for the later stages of labor.

## ANTERIOR CERVICAL LIP

An anterior cervical lip may develop during dilation in first stage labor. Place the mother upright if she has been prone, or lying on one side then the other if she has been upright. Relieve swelling by icing the lip and/or administering homeopathic Sepia 200C and Arnica 200C. Once dilation is nearly complete, the lip can be managed by placing the fingers on the lip where it touches the fetal head and massaging the lip back over the fetal head above the inferior border of the pubic symphysis. The lip should be held in place until the next contraction when the woman is asked to push down. The fingers are allowed to be pushed down and out while the fetal head presses against the inferior border. When the lip remains in the new position over the fetal head, the fingers can be removed. It may be helpful to have the mother half squatting during this maneuver.

## POSTERIOR ASYNCLITISM

### *MANUAL INTERNAL ROTATION*

Internal exam confirms the position of the fetal head. Disengage the head by placing fingers on either side of the sagittal suture and lightly pressing upward on the parietal bones. The mother then fully reclines with an assistant next to her on the side of the fetal back, facing the midwife. Steady, even pressure on the bony edge of the anterior fontanelle is used to rotate it to a transverse position. The fontanelle is pressed toward the vaginal side wall. The posterior fontanelle is then caught and rotated to the anterior while the assistant presses the fetal body to the anterior with mother turning in the direction of fontanelle rotation. The mother should then sit upright and stand with a forward leaning position to secure the fetal position. Without an assistant the mother assumes knees-chest position. If the fetus reverts to the previous position, make another attempt. Do not use force.

### *MATERNAL POSITIONAL CHANGES OR EXERCISES*

Posterior asynclitism, a condition where the posterior parietal bone presents at the cervix, may be managed for repositioning in several ways. The mother can try to duck-walk to open the pelvis and encourage the fetus to reposition. Climbing stairs two at a time produces the same effect. Another method is a hip twist and lift where the mother alternates throwing a hip and leg forward then bending and straightening the leg, or performing a lunge by placing a leg on a chair seat and leaning into a lunge position with each contraction. Finding a way to shake the mother, as in a rough car ride, or using a rebozo beneath the hips of a supine mother to rock the hips quickly from side to side may also achieve a repositioning of the fetal head.

### Techniques Ineffective in Preserving an Intact Perineum

The least effective techniques massage or place pressure on the perineum prior to crowning. In some instances, the technique creates conditions favorable to a tear or laceration. This includes "ironing out" the perineum by sweeping the fingers from side to side within the vaginal vault using pressure on the posterior vaginal wall ahead of the crown. This may bruise the tissue which then may tear. Perineal massage with warmed oils or lubricants is thought to increase circulation and relax the perineum, but creates a tendency to lacerate. A third technique supports the perineum at the time of birth by bracing the perineal body with the hand, but this tends to block the fetal head from descending properly and can force the tissue from the midline, both conditions may cause tearing. The ironing and massaging techniques are also known to be irritating and distracting to some women.

### Elevator Pelvic Floor Exercise

Tearing and lacerations may be decreased or prevented if the mother has vaginal muscle control. The "elevator" exercise teaches this control. The pelvic floor muscles pull up as if they were part of an elevator. The elevator stops at the first, second, third, fourth, and fifth floors. At each point hold the pelvic muscles momentarily. Once the "fifth floor" is reached, hold the muscles 30 seconds and descend the elevator, pausing at each floor and stopping at the "sub-basement" where birth takes place.

Another exercise to teach muscle control strengthens the bulbocavernosus muscle by making snapping movements low in the vagina near the introitus. An alternate approach is to contract first the bulbocavernosus muscle, then the transverse perineal muscle, then the vaginal canal, and finally the levator ani. Once all the layers are contracted, the muscles are held briefly and then released in the opposite order.

### Preserving an Intact Perineum

Maternal self-control is the best way to preserve the perineum no matter the method used. Warm compresses applied to the perineum increase circulation in the local area and relax the muscles, decreasing the risk of tearing. Prenatal digital stretching, while not proven to be protective of the perineum, can familiarize the mother with the sensation of pressure in that area, relieving anxiety about tearing or episiotomy. Perineal support can be performed by placing the thumb and the middle finger in the left and right groin leaving a slight gap between the hand and the perineum. Inward pressure is applied with the finger and thumb to increase the flexibility of the perineum without blocking the head. A third technique, which is mandatory in lithotomy and dorsal birth positions to prevent tearing, is to control the fetal head by applying pressure against it to keep it flexed then allowing gradual extension as the perineum stretches.

### When to Encourage Pushing

In most instances it is best to wait until the urge to push overcomes the mother as the body is most likely to be prepared for this activity. It has been found that encouraging pushing before the desire to do so exerts itself often leads to fetal bradycardia, an increased need for episiotomies, and an increased need for fetal resuscitation. However, in certain circumstances, aggressive pushing may be required. In a situation where the fetus is crashing and must be birthed quickly to be resuscitated, you must have the mother push to help speed delivery. These circumstances also often require you to perform an episiotomy now or extensive suture repair later.

## Indicators of Imminent Birth

There is often a period of time, typically about an hour, between stage one and stage two labor in which the mother should be encouraged to rest. Stage two labor is usually signaled by an intense desire to push, meaning that the fetal head has descended to the perineal floor. Delivery is approaching when rectal bulging, perineal bulging, and progressive visibility of the fetal head at the vaginal introitus are observed. The mother may express the desire to use the bathroom. If she indicates the reason is she feels a bowel movement coming, it is likely the birth is imminent. A very definite indication that birth has arrived is if the mother vocalizes that her baby is coming. It is unwise not to listen to her.

## Abnormal Fetal Heart Tones

Any nonreassuring fetal heart tone that cannot be attributed to narcotic administration or fails to resolve with in utero rescusitation efforts must be reported to the consulting physician immediately.

Management consists of the following steps in order:

- Rule out a prolapsed umbilical cord. If prolapse is found, perform emergency deliver procedures
- Determine rapid descent of the head
- Determine length of time to birth
- Stimulate fetal scalp
- Monitor the fetus internally if needed
- IV hydration without glucose
- Discontinue any oxytocin augmentation
- Administer oxygen at 8 to 10 L/min (this is ineffective if cord compression is complete)
- Stimulate scalp, acoustic, or abdominal fetal stimulation. If no response, obtain fetal scalp blood sample
- Administer tocolytic therapy without delaying intervention
- Amnioinfusion
- Prepare for caesarian section if FHR continues to worsen

As these steps are carried out, the mother and support partner(s) must be kept fully informed of the seriousness of the situation.

## Non-Emergency Management of Nonreassuring FHR Patterns or FHT

Nonreassuring FHR patterns may not be emergency situations. If the fetus has had normal FHR patterns immediately prior to developing an abnormal pattern and it is due to a short duration of decreased variability less than 60 minutes without decelerations, or multiple mild or moderate decelerations with quick return to baseline and variability, or transient tachycardia, management consists of:

- Positioning the mother on her side
- Determining hydration needs and augmenting with IV fluids without glucose
- Considering fetal sleep cycle, oligohydramnios, narcotic administration
- Fetal scalp or acoustic stimulation

- Intermittent auscultation or electronic fetal monitoring
- Internal fetal scalp electrode for monitoring and stimulation

If unchanged notify the consulting physician.

## Factors That Contribute to Nonreassuring FHT

Factors to consider when diagnosing nonreassuring fetal heart tones or fetal heart rate patterns are as follows:

- Administration of narcotic to mother
- Maternal conditions that contribute to uteroplacental insufficiency: diabetes, lupus erythematosus, hypertension, preeclampsia
- Fetal conditions that contribute these abnormalities: postdates, oligohydramnios, postdates, IUGR
- Differential diagnosis of the FHR pattern itself
- Any tachycardia and/or decreased variability
- Success of corrective attempts
- Acid-base status of the fetus
- Whether meconium is present
- Gestational age
- Expected time to birth
- Availability of emergency medical intervention

## Umbilical Cord Prolapse

When a cord prolapse occurs:

- You place your entire hand into the vagina to hold the presenting part off the cord at the pelvic inlet
- The cord MUST NOT be replaced. This may cause cord spasm or further compression
- Summon assistance, inform the mother and secure her cooperation
- Send STAT notification to the consulting physician
- Have other helpers place the mother in Trendelenberg or knee-chest to keep the fetus off the pelvic inlet
- Wrap any cord protruding through the vagina in gauze soaked with warm saline
- Perform an emergency caesarian section is performed

Assess the FHT with ultrasound, fetoscope or Dopplar. Cord pulsations will not be a reliable indicator of fetal health. Your hand must remain in the vagina supporting the presenting part until the fetus is delivered.

### *Types and Causes of Umbilical Cord Prolapse*

Frank cord prolapse: the cord has protruded through the cervix.

Occult cord prolapse: the cord lays aside the presenting part but does not protrude through the cervix.

Umbilical cord prolapse is at high risk when:

- membranes rupture and fetus is in breech, compound presentation, transverse lie, second born twin, or a small fetus weighing less than 2000 grams
- membranes are ruptured and the presenting part is an unengaged head, unengaged breech, footling breech, compound presentation, or shoulder and an enema is administered
- An amniotomy is performed and the head is unengaged, there is a compound presentation, a non-cephalic presentation, or a small fetus with a presenting part that does not fill the pelvis
- A vaginal exam is performed that ruptures the membranes with the membranes bulging, and an unengaged head, a non-cephalic presentation, or a compound presentation
- There is SROM with unengaged head, non-cephalic presentation, or compound presentation
- A fetal assessment or obstetric intervention disturbs the vertex

### *Observing for and Differential Diagnosis of Umbilical Cord Prolapse*

Whenever the membranes rupture, the FHT must be assessed and a vaginal exam performed to check for a prolapsed cord. The examiner must feel around the presenting part, in the vagina, at the intersection of the presenting part and the external cervical os, each of the vaginal fornices, and palpate the thinned lower uterus. Occasionally the midwife will be asked to see a mother who has "something coming out between her legs". A vaginal exam will reveal whether it is a cord, a mucus plug, or a prolapsed foot or arm.

## Nuchal Cord

During the birthing process, the hand that receives the head slides down the baby's upper back and sweeps side to side to feel for the presence of an umbilical cord near the head. If present and loose, slip it over the baby's head. If the cord is too tight for the head but is not tight around the neck, slip the cord over the shoulders and allow the body to birth through it. If it is too tight to maneuver over the shoulders but can be loosened a little, the shoulders should be slowly delivered without moving the cord, and then the baby's neck is flexed so the face is toward the mother's thigh. The head is kept near the perineum as the body is delivered (somersault). The cord is then unwrapped. If the cord is tight, the mother must be told to pant while the cord is immediately clamped, cut and unwound before delivery of the body.

## Face and Brow Presentation

The consulting physician should be notified once a diagnosis of face presentation has been made by abdominal palpation and pelvic examination. Do not apply an electrode for internal monitoring because fetal eye damage may result. Reassess the pelvic capacity for CPD. If the fetus assumes direct mentum posterior position during rotation, notify the consulting physician. To deliver the head, apply pressure to the brow until the chin is born. Once the chin and the rest of the head are born, complete the delivery normally. Assess and treat the infant for any edema of the trachea, nose, and mouth. Reassure the parents any swelling and facial distortion will reverse in a few days.

Brow presentation, unless transitory prior to face presentation, will cause the largest diametrical portion of the head to present which is nearly always too large for the pelvic outlet. A caesarian section is typically required.

## Rules and Steps in Delivering a Multiple Birth

An unexpected multiple birth must never be due to a failure by the attending midwife to diagnose multiple gestation during the prenatal period. Contact emergency services even though transport may not be possible before delivery. Limit medications during labor since the fetuses are likely preterm or small for gestational age and less able to withstand the effects. Prepare the mother as much as possible for medical management, including placing an IV and drawing blood for type and crossmatch. Deliver the first fetus according to its presentation and position. Quickly clamp and cut the cord to prevent the possibility of the other fetus(es) bleeding out through the cord. An assistant should maneuver the remaining fetus into position and place it into the true pelvis. Carefully monitor the remaining fetus' heart tones and watch the vagina for bleeding. The second fetus should deliver 3 to 15 minutes after the first. Once the remaining fetus is in place, rupture the membranes. If contractions do not continue, medication may be required to stimulate delivery.

## Membranes Presenting at Birth

Typically, if the membranes are bulging from the vagina they are ruptured by the descent of the head and the waters flow out ahead of the baby. Occasionally the rupture occurs higher up and the membranes envelop the face as it is born, called "delivery in the caul". This is a breathing obstruction that must be corrected immediately. A finger must be hooked into the membrane below the chin and the membrane peeled away. This issue can be avoided if the midwife and mother both agree to artificially rupture the membrane if it presents in this manner. Cultural sensitivity must be used as this condition is seen in some cultures as "good luck". The midwife should have a good sense of how the family sees such a presentation.

## Shoulder Dystocia

Shoulder dystocia is defined as a failure of the shoulders to spontaneously birth after the head delivers. The anterior shoulder is caught behind or on the pubic symphysis and the posterior shoulder is in the sacral hollow or above the sacral promontory. Any traction further compacts the anterior shoulder and obstructs the delivery of the rest of the body. The incidence of shoulder dystocia is around 0.37% to 1.1%.

Risk increases with:

- Post-term pregnancy
- high parity
- maternal obesity
- maternal age over 35
- maternal diabetes
- gestational diabetes
- fetal macrosomia
- oxytocin induction
- prolonged labor
- operative deliveries
- prolonged second stage labor

If the delivery is initially uncomplicated but the head birthed slowly with problems in delivering the chin over the perineum, shoulder dystocia may be implicated. The head may appear to be receding back into the vagina as reverse traction ensues. If normal maneuvers to birth the baby fail, shoulder dystocia is diagnosed.

## Moderate Shoulder Dystocia

Mobilize the emergency plan. Tell the mother the problem, state that the solution will be painful, and that she must not push. Place her in McRobert's maneuver (exaggerated lithotomy). Knee-chest is the same position only upside down. The fetal shoulders are rotated into the oblique position. DO NOT MOVE THE HEAD. One hand is placed on one side of the fetal chest, the other behind the opposite shoulder blade; as much force as necessary is used to rotate the body. The assistant applies suprapubic pressure in the direction you specify while you press downward and outward on the side of the head. Fundal pressure should never be given.

If the baby is still not delivered, catheterize the mother, determine the need for an episiotomy, and perform a vaginal exam for short cord, enlarged fetal thorax or abdomen. The baby is then delivered on a renewed attempt from McRobert's maneuver.

## Severe Shoulder Dystocia

### *Delivering the Posterior Arm*

In severe shoulder dystocia rotation of the fetal shoulders and delivery using McRobert's maneuver has failed. Delivering the posterior arm can be attempted before or after the corkscrew maneuver. You place your entire hand into the vagina and follow the fetal arm to the elbow and forearm. Flex the arm by pressing the antecubital space and bringing it across the fetal abdomen and chest in the normal range of motion until the hand can be grasped and the arm delivered. Do not hook the fingers into the axilla or armpit. Delivery is completed using McRobert's maneuver, suprapubic pressure, and downward and outward pressure on the fetal head. If delivery is still not possible, the fetus can be rotated 180 degrees in the corkscrew maneuver and delivery attempted again. Nearly all severe shoulder dystocias are delivered by one or both of these methods. A last resort if they fail is to fracture the fetal clavicle or use the Zavanelli maneuver.

## Corkscrew Maneuver

In severe shoulder dystocia fetal shoulder rotation and delivery using McRobert's maneuver have failed. Place the hands on the fetal chest and back as in a typical rotation procedure but the fetus is rotated 180 degrees one direction, then 180 degrees the opposite direction until the baby is "screwed out". The fetus should be rotated so the back is rotated anteriorly. It is most effective to change hand positions at 90 degrees and continue the rotation to the full 180 degrees. Three to four complete rotations should be attempted before abandoning this maneuver. This maneuver can be performed before or after delivering the posterior arm. Nearly all severe shoulder dystocias are delivered by one or both of these methods. A last resort if they fail is to fracture the fetal clavicle or use the Zavanelli maneuver.

## Quiet Catastrophic Uterine Rupture

In quiet uterine rupture, there may or may not be maternal vomiting; there may be increased abdominal tenderness, hypotonic uterine contractions, severe suprapubic pain, lack of labor progress from the time of rupture, and maternal syncope. Later hematuria, slight pain, vaginal bleeding, and shock will occur. Contractions may be ineffective or cease and fetal heart tones are not evident. All of these signs may also be seen in placental abruption. Bleeding into the peritoneum may cause the diaphragm to become irritated and pain to be felt in the chest in imitation of amniotic fluid or pulmonary embolism. Emergency services and the consulting physician should be notified immediately and two IV routes placed, one for blood transfusion and one for electrolyte solution. Oxygen must be administered and transport obtained. It is likely a hysterectomy will result.

## Types of Uterine Rupture

There are two types of uterine rupture.

- Catastrophic uterine rupture involves the old incision separating completely. The fetal membranes rupture; part, or all, of the fetus extrudes into the peritoneal cavity; and hemorrhage is significant. The first sign of catastrophic rupture is fetal bradycardia; any change in FHT, especially recurrent late decelerations and which are not relieved by any action, may indicate a rupture is imminent. The most serious sign is recurrent late decelerations followed by prolonged decelerations and terminal bradycardia.

  In dramatic rupture, the mother feels a sharp, shooting abdominal pain at the peak of a contraction. The presenting part is now movable, a loss of station or repositioning is apparent, fetal parts are easily palpated, fetal movements are violent and then cease, the contracted uterus is felt beside the fetus. Maternal shock may occur.

- Atraumatic dehiscence is where the old scar does not separate along the entire length, the fetal membranes do not rupture, the fetus does not extrude into the peritoneal cavity, and there is little to no bleeding

## Amniotic Fluid Embolism

Maternal symptoms are:

- extreme shortness of breath, gasping, hypoxia
- significant decrease in blood pressure
- depressed cardiac function
- seizures
- DIC (Disseminated Intravascular Coagulation)

Typically occurring during hard labor, it is caused when amniotic fluid or fetal cells enter the mother's bloodstream. Although this is a rare complication maternal mortality rate is 60-80%. The mother must be transported to a hospital immediately. If the baby is delivered within 15 minutes of embolic occurrence, there is a 67% chance of intact survival of the baby. Maternal management includes treatment for shock, CPR with oxygen, and an IV. If the birth is complete, bimanual compression helps prevent bleed-out. The mother should then be transported to the hospital. At this time there is no known cause of amniotic fluid embolism although it is thought that abortion, amniocentesis, amnioinfusion, or hyperstimulation of the uterus with an oxytocic may cause this complication.

## Stillbirth and Neonatal Death

The coroner must be notified of any stillborn weighing 500 grams or more. An autopsy is at the discretion of the coroner. If it can established that the baby has been dead for a period of time, the autopsy may be optional. The coroner releases the body to the funeral home chosen by the parents and signs the death certificate. The midwife should plan to spend time with the parents for the first weeks. After allowing time for grieving, the parents should be encouraged to prepare a memorial such as a chronicle of the birth and death, or a scrapbook. The basic phases of grieving should be discussed with the parents and the appropriate referrals to support groups and written materials on speaking to children and siblings about death should be given.

## APGAR Scoring System

The APGAR score is used for standardized assessment for the need for resuscitation of the newborn. Someone other than the midwife should perform the APGAR scoring and the person who does the scoring should be the one to chart it. This prevents errors. The APGAR score takes into account the newborn's heart rate, respiratory effort, muscle tone, reflex irritability, and color, assigning each a score according to various characteristics of these factors. The APGAR score is always performed at 1 and 5 minutes and again at 10 minutes if previous scores are nonreassuring. A healthy newborn will have a score of 7 to 10 at one and five minutes. A score of less than 3 is associated with the highest mortality during the first 28 days of life no matter the gestational age. If a low APGAR score is still determined after 10 to 20 minutes there is a high risk of cerebral palsy developing.

### First Minute After Birth

Immediately establish a clear airway by holding the infant so the head is below the body, wipe the face and head, and clean fluid from the nose and mouth. Suction the nasal and oral cavities. Keep the infant warm, preferably on the mother's abdomen with a cap placed on its head and covered with a blanket. Show the infant to the mother and partner if they have not seen it. Clamp and cut the cord. Examine the infant for visible anomalies and congenital abnormalities. Assign the 1 minute APGAR score. Perform the final cord cutting.

### Primary and Secondary Apnea

Primary apnea and secondary apnea are the two categories of neonatal depression.

Primary apnea is a condition in which the infant has not been hypoxic for long, but is already attempting to breathe more rapidly in utero to compensate. Stimulation, blow-by oxygen, or a few breaths of mouth to mouth resuscitation should revive this infant.

Secondary apnea is a condition in an infant who has been hypoxic for much longer than above and making a second attempt in utero to breathe more rapidly without succeeding in restoring oxygen levels. This infant will not attempt to breathe again on its own. Immediate ventilation is required via mouth-to-mouth or bag-mask to reverse acidosis caused by hypoxia. The baby's color, muscle tone, and respiratory effort guide the choice of resuscitation technique. The baby is suctioned, then warmed and stimulated by massaging it from the base of the spine up the back. The mother's voice may encourage a rise in oxygen level.

## TTN

Transient tachypnea of the newborn (TTN) is a temporary condition in which the newborn has abnormally rapid breathing. This occurs in 1-2% of newborns. TTN is also called "wet lungs" or type II respiratory distress syndrome. Infants born to mothers who smoked during pregnancy or had diabetes and infants small for their gestational age are at higher risk for this condition. Normal newborn breathing rates are 40-60 breaths per minute. TTN may increase these rates to 120 breaths per minute. TTN is caused by delayed absorption of fetal lung fluid and is a condition that will often resolve itself within 24-72 hours. However, if it is accompanied by respiratory distress syndrome, meconium aspiration, sepsis or any sign of respiratory problems the baby must see the pediatrician immediately. Once TTN resolves, the infant is at no higher risk of other respiratory illness than any other newborn.

### Circumoral Cyanosis and Central Cyanosis

According to Tabor's Cyclopedic Medical Dictionary, 20th edition, the terms are synonymous. Central (circumoral) cyanosis is defined as a bluish discoloration of the mucous membranes of the mouth which indicates hypoxemia and respiratory failure. In Varney's Midwifery 4th edition, central cyanosis is used to refer to a bluish discoloration of not only the oral mucous membranes, but the lips, tongue, and trunk. In any case, cyanosis is a sign of respiratory distress or compromise. Cyanosis, along with grunting, nasal flaring, and retractions of the intercostal muscles, are all indicators of respiratory compromise. Retraction of the sternum indicates severe respiratory compromise. Grunting typically indicates air trapped within a lung.

## Newborn Resuscitation

First and foremost, the airway must be cleared. Without a clear airway all other efforts will be futile. Once an airway has been established, give the newborn a few breaths by way of a pocket mask or positive pressure ventilation (PPV) while awaiting oxygen. Once spontaneous respiration is in evidence, PPV may be stopped and free flow oxygen given if color is still bluish. If spontaneous respiration does not commence, PPV using 5 to 10 L/min of oxygen at the rate of 40 to 60 respirations per minute through a resuscitation bag and mask should be performed. PPV should pause every 30 seconds to check for spontaneous respiration.

## Meconium Aspiration

Infants with moderate to heavy meconium at birth may develop respiratory problems. If lung obstruction is heard or the baby's respiration is too rapid, the baby should be observed for other signs of respiratory distress syndrome:

- nasal flaring
- grunting upon exhalation
- retractions of the chest and abdomen
- cyanosis

If any of these signs are observed, blow-by oxygen should be administered and the baby immediately transported to the hospital with notification of pediatric support. If none of these signs is observed, the baby's breathing may be made easier by using steam to loosen any congestion. In addition, apply percussion using two or three fingertips to tap sharply in each lung quadrant while the baby rests on your lap head down. If the congestion remains unresolved, the pediatrician should be notified. Otherwise, the baby may be observed overnight by the parents for further problems.

## Umbilical Cord

The umbilical cord is typically clamped using two clamps with room between for cutting. Prior to placing the second clamp the cord can be stripped to remove blood from the area where the cord will be cut. This will prevent spraying of blood from the cord. The clamp must not be allowed to dangle and place pressure on the placenta. In term infants there is no evidence that waiting for the cord to stop pulsing to cut it has any effect on the health of the newborn. Premature newborns may benefit from being held in a warm blanket below the placenta to receive the additional blood prior to cutting the cord. It also has not been shown that the cord stump requires anything other than water for cleaning unless signs of infection are present. Blood from the cord is collected for typing and direct Coombs.

## New Ballard Scale

The New Ballard Scale (NBS) can accurately date the gestational age of a newborn down to 20 weeks plus or minus 2 weeks. The scale confers scores on various observable abilities and characteristics of the newborn and uses the score to establish the gestational age. The characteristics and abilities include posture, "square window" which measures flexion of the hand, arm recoil, popliteal angle, the scarf sign, and the heel to toe maneuver. The observations also include the amount of lanugo on the back, the presence of cartilage in the pinna of the ear, and an assessment of breast tissue, as well as other physical characteristics. The gestational age assessment is applied by using it to categorize the newborn, firstly as preterm (<38 weeks), term (38-42 weeks), and post-term (>42 weeks), then used in conjunction with birth weight. The newborn is further categorized as small for gestational age (SGA), appropriate for gestational age (AGA), and large for gestational age (LGA).

## Third Stage Labor

The uterus is substantially decreased in size after the birth of the newborn. The placenta grows thicker to adapt to the decreased space but the area of attachment between placenta and uterus cannot shrink and the placenta detaches from the uterine wall. A hematoma forms and helps complete the separation. The placenta then descends into the lower uterus or upper vagina causing bleeding, increased visible umbilical cord length, changed uterine shape, and allowing the uterus to rise in the abdomen through uterine displacement. The uterus becomes globular. As the cord lengthens the mother may feel the placenta in the vaginal vault. Place the mother in a squat if possible to deliver the placenta. The membranes should follow.

## Placental Separation in Third Stage Labor

If the cord has been cut, the clamp can be observed to move downward as the placenta detaches in the third stage of labor. Cord blood, if needed, must be collected before separation occurs. Excessive bleeding should be noted as there should be minimal blood loss until placental separation. In rare cases, the placenta only separates in the center with outer margins attached. The uterus grows larger and blood filled; the mother can go into shock. Guarding the uterus, with a hand resting on the fundus as soon as birth occurs and leaving it there until placental delivery helps rule out such a separation. The fundus should not be prodded or massaged as this could cause partial separation and hemorrhage.

## Facilitating Delivery of the Placenta

The placenta typically delivers around 30 minutes after birth, occasionally as much as 60 minutes. Breast-feeding or other form of nipple stimulation causes or enhances uterine contractions which in turn speed placental separation and delivery. Once the placenta is at the cervical os or in the vagina and the uterus has completely contracted, controlled cord traction may be used. Care must be taken with this maneuver to prevent uterine inversion which may prove fatal to the mother. The uterus is held in place with the edge of a hand pressing inward and upward just above the pubic bone. Traction is gently applied to the cord first downward then outward as in the birth of the infant. The mother should push while this it performed. The membranes may not follow immediately and may need to be teased out. When the mother delivers in a squat this is rarely an issue. The placenta should be gently delivered a short distance into a container otherwise any adherent membranes may tear and separate.

## Angelica and Shepherd's Purse

Angelica and Shepherd's Purse, in tincture form, are both helpful herbal remedies for delayed or slow placental delivery or postpartum blood loss. Angelica is used to facilitate uterine contractions for placental delivery "like an angel". A few drops are placed under the mother's tongue. It may also be used for partial placental separation and to ensure complete delivery. Shepherd's Purse is given after placental delivery to facilitate clotting so it is important the placenta be completely delivered prior to administration (along with Blue Cohosh) to cause uterine contractions to expel excess clots and reduce bleeding. Another herbal remedy that is said to facilitate placental delivery is *Glechoma hederacea*, or Ground Ivy Herb, administered as a tincture. The administration of raspberry leaf infusion during labor is helpful for ensuring uterine contractual efficiency.

## Characteristics Examined After Delivery

The following characteristics of the cord, membranes, and placenta are inspected for completeness and health. The umbilical cord: There should be three cord vessels, two arteries and a vein. The presence of only two vessels may indicate a non-visible fetal anomaly. It should also be inspected for knots, tumors, cysts, edema and hematomas. The volume of Wharton's jelly should also be noted along with the location of cord insertion (eccentric, marginal, or central). The membranes: The membranes are inspected for completeness and succenturiate lobes, blood vessels, or defects. The placenta: The placenta is observed for meconium staining and calcifications. The fetal side is observed for cysts, a determination of extrachorial placenta, and missing or intact succenturiate lobe. The maternal side is observed for infarcts and intactness such as missing colydon.

The placenta is often weighed and the umbilical cord measured, especially if they are abnormally small or large.

## Assessing the Delivered Placenta

"Dirty Duncan" refers to a placenta that delivers with the meaty maternal side presenting. This occurs when the placenta separates along the edges and is often found in placentas that implanted low in the uterus. "Shiny Schultz" refers to the placenta that presents the fetal side with shiny membranes upon delivery. This occurs when the placenta begins separation in the center.

## Trickle Bleed After Placenta Delivery

Once the placenta has been delivered, the uterus is checked for complete contraction. A quick, firm massage will facilitate the expulsion of any remaining clots. If the mother is in a squat the massage is not necessary. If the uterus continues to feel soft or asymmetrical, or if excess bleeding is occurring, firm massage, nipple stimulation (especially breastfeeding) and/or administration of Shepherd's Purse and blue Cohosh tinctures can facilitate further contractions. The mother's bladder should be checked for distention as this can also keep the uterus from full contraction. Bleeding may also be caused by retained placental fragments. An inspection of the placenta for completeness will answer this question. Any retained fragments must be removed before bleeding can be controlled. Neither massage nor pitocin will help in this case.

## Fundal Massage, and External and Internal Bimanual Compression

Fundal massage is generally the first response to uterine atony. It is an attempt to cause the uterus to contract itself and thereby staunch bleeding. If this is unsuccessful or bleeding is severe, you must manually contract or compress the uterus. This can be done externally by lifting the uterus through the abdominal wall and squeezing it between both hands. Internal bimanual compression involves placing one hand inside the vagina, palmar surface up and fisted. The other hand is pushed deeply into the abdomen and behind the uterus. The uterus is then compressed between the external hand and the internal fist. This compresses internal uterine vessels and causes the uterus to contract.

## Fourth Stage Intrauterine Exploration

Fourth stage intrauterine exploration is performed to ensure no clots, retained placental fragments, or membranes are left in the uterus which may be inhibiting the complete contraction of the uterus or causing bleeding. A gauze pad is wrapped around the forefinger of a gloved hand. This hand is placed entirely inside the uterus. The back of the hand is placed against the uterine wall. The other hand is placed on the abdomen at the same area as the internal hand. The uterus is swept and anything on the gauze pad is identified. The uterus can then be swept a second time with a new gauze if needed. Oxytocin and/or Methergine are administered to promote uterine contractions. Herbal remedies such as Shepherd's Purse and blue Cohosh may also be used. In some cases, the mother can stop the bleeding by focusing on the problem, tightening the uterus and taking control of her body.

### Uterine Consistency After Delivery

Uterine tone is assessed in the fourth stage of labor, after the delivery of the placenta. The flow of lochia is also assessed at this time. Assessment is by fundal massage in which the lower uterus is stabilized at the symphysis pubis with one hand and the entire fundus is quickly, gently, and firmly massaged with the other. If the uterus is fully contracted, there will be no increased lochial flow during massage. If the uterus is relaxed and boggy, the lochial flow will increase, sometimes significantly. If uterine contractions are facilitated this issue will not occur. Breastfeeding or other nipple stimulation will help keep the uterus contracted as will frequent light uterine massage. The mother should be taught to perform light uterine massage and to check her lochia regularly for the first 24 to 48 hours after birth.

### Immediate Postpartum Hemorrhage

Most immediate postpartum hemorrhages are caused by:

- incomplete delivery of the placenta or uterine atony which may be due to an overdistended uterus
- oxytocin induction or augmentation
- uterine relaxing medications
- grand multiparity
- rapid labor and delivery
- history of uterine atony or postpartum hemorrhage
- prolonged first or second stage labor

Other causes include cervical lacerations, extensive vaginal or perineal lacerations, and laceration of the lower uterus/uterine rupture, which is rare.

Previously known abnormal conditions can also result in this type of hemorrhage: placenta previa, caesarian section, placental abruption, retention of a dead fetus, or operative procedures. If a client has two or more risk factors for uterine atony, the birth should be in a hospital. Other anticipatory activities include the readiness of medications and staff for such an event.

### Third Stage Hemorrhage

Third stage hemorrhage is caused by partial placental separation which in turn is often caused by uterine massage prior to placental delivery. While the placenta may become partially separate during delivery, the condition is usually short lived, but separation due to medical mismanagement almost always causes hemorrhage. If hemorrhaging in the third stage occurs, someone other than the midwife should immediately call the consulting physician and emergency services. Thoroughly massage the uterus to try to complete the placental separation. Place an IV with Ringer's Lactate and draw blood for a type and crossmatch. Watch the mother and manage signs of shock. Catheterize her unless her bladder is known to be empty. Manually separate and deliver the placenta if it has not already been. If you are unable to do so and emergency services have not yet arrived, an oxytocin solution that causes intermittent contractions should be given to contract the uterus and cervix ONLY IF ABSOLUTELY NECESSARY.

## Post-Partum Hemorrhage

There are three elements to avoiding post-partum hemorrhage:

- Good nutrition and supplements
- Familiarity with the mother
- Delivery of the placenta without urgency

With proper nutrition the mother will maintain hemostasis more readily. Certain supplements such as liquid chlorophyll, red raspberry and nettles or tincture of nettles, yellowdock, alfalfa and red raspberry as well as multivitamins can keep nutritional levels at optimum.

Delivery of the placenta should not be rushed but taken in its own time so that the intervillous spaces can contract and control blood flow.

Familiarity with the mother allows you to be aware of the mother's diet and previous birth experiences. It also means that all recent lab results have been obtained and checked, especially the hemoglobin, hematocrit, and platelet count.

### Emergency Measures for Uncontrolled Postpartum Hemorrhage

If all steps have been taken to control postpartum hemorrhage including medications, bimanual compression, and intrauterine exploration, the emergency backup plan must be activated. The consulting physician should have already been notified. Patent IV catheters should be in place for further medication use or for blood transfusion. If not already obtained, a blood sample for type and crossmatch should be drawn. If the mother is going into shock as observed by decreasing blood pressure, rapid pulse and respirations, and cold, clammy skin, she should be placed in Trendelenberg, covered with blankets, and given oxygen and blood. The mother is then maintained until arrival of the physician.

### Bladder Distension After Delivery

Bladder distension is diagnosed when the uterus is assessed during the so-called fourth stage of labor, or the stage after the placenta is delivered. Uterine assessment by abdominal palpation will reveal the uterus above and, typically, to the right of the umbilicus. This indicates a full bladder which can prevent the uterus from contracting and increased bleeding will occur. It is also a risk for bladder infection. The bladder may develop hypotonicity which leads to the loss of the urge to urinate. The mother should be encouraged to urinate. If she is unable to do so after repeated attempts, she should be catheterized to empty the bladder. Catheterization should not be the first choice due to the discomfort it causes to the mother and the increased potential for infection.

### Cervix, Vagina, and Perineum Assessment Immediately Postpartum

The cervix is assessed only if a steady flow or trickle of bright red blood from the vagina is observed, or if there was rapid labor, cervical manipulation during labor, pushing before dilation was complete, or a traumatic or instrument delivery. Otherwise, the cervix does not require assessment which can be painful to the mother. The lower vagina, periurethral areas, and the perineum are assessed for lacerations and torn blood vessels, including determination of the need to repair; bruising; and hematoma. Episiotomies are assessed for depth and extensions. The perianal area is assessed for hemorrhoids and skin tears. Episiotomy extensions into the rectal area are also checked. Hemorrhoids can be treated with ice packs, astringents, and/or analgesic sprays.

## Terms

Cystocele: a swelling of the vaginal tissues at the opening of the vagina near the urethra. This is caused by weakening and straining of the muscles of the vaginal vault.

Rectocele: a swelling of the vaginal tissues at the opening of the vagina near the perineum. This is caused by weakening or straining of the pelvic floor muscles.

Hematoma: An asymmetrical, painful swelling of the perineal area caused by soft tissue trauma in second stage labor and a tissue repair that has not contained or stopped bleeding vessels below the skin or mucosal surfaces. The resultant pooling of blood can allow bacterial growth, infection and repair breakdown, and failure of the tissues to close. This may result in the need for reconstructive surgery.

## Perineal Tears

Unless the birth is in water, one technique for preventing tears in the perineum is application of hot compresses. Such compresses stimulate blood circulation. They also relieve some of the burning felt by the mother when the perineum is stretched to its fullest. In addition to these, the compress promotes relaxation which in turn helps the mother to continue the birth process more easily. To make the compresses, sterile gauze pads or clean washcloths are soaked in hot water with an antiseptic agent added. The pad is pressed onto the perineum and is most useful if the perineum begins to blanch. If the pressure of the descending head causes the mother to pass fecal matter, it should be wiped away with a tissue. If the compress becomes contaminated, it should be exchanged for a clean one.

## First, Second, Third, and Fourth Degree Lacerations

Degree of laceration/tissues involved:

- First degree/vaginal mucosa, posterior fourchette, and perineal skin
- Second degree/vaginal mucosa, posterior fourchette, perineal skin and perineal muscles
- Third degree/vaginal mucosa, posterior fourchette, perineal skin, perineal muscles, and external anal sphincter
- Fourth degree/vaginal mucosa, posterior fourchette, perineal skin, perineal muscles, external anal sphincter, and anterior rectal wall

When determining the repair of lacerations, consideration must be given to the severity of the laceration and whether a repair is truly necessary. Some first degree lacerations do not require repair, such as vaginal abrasions, some perineal lacerations, or minor tears of the bulbous cavernosus. Direct pressure can be enough to staunch bleeding. Others can be repaired using various suture techniques. Second degree lacerations require sutures but are often more ragged and it is difficult to match the tissues together. Sutures must be placed accordingly. Third degree lacerations include extensions of a midline episiotomy or a sphincterotomy. Identification of the degree of laceration in third and fourth degree lacerations prior to suturing is crucial.

## Basic Suture Principles

- Close all lacerations in layers – muscle, fascia, skin. This will eliminate tension in a particular area.
- Dead spaces between layers should be eliminated. If they are not, oozing can occur and a hematoma may form which is a risk for infection.
- The suture should not be too tight or circulation will be impaired. Allowances must be made for the possibility of swelling.

- Using too many stitches can also result in circulatory impairment.
- Landmarks must be checked very carefully and repeatedly. If enough time has passed before the sutures are made swelling may confuse the issue.
- Sutures should have greater depth than width.
- Never clamp the suture with the needle holder because it may break at the site.
- If possible, have an assistant handy to cut sutures as they are placed to prevent the person performing the suture from the need to exchange instruments.

## Postpartum Perineal Care

It has been found that the amount of information presented to a new mother should be kept to the minimum necessary for good self and newborn care in the immediate postpartum and puerperium. Instruct the mother to maintain good hand-washing practices, to rinse the perineal area with warm water while eliminating and voiding, to make certain to wipe front to back, and to pat the incision rather than rub it. In addition, share information regarding treatment of discomfort and encourage the mother to perform Kegel exercises to increase tone. Sitz baths, which can include herbs such as Comfrey leaf, Yarrow, Rosemary, Golden Seal, Oak bark, Witch hazel, Sea Grape bark, and Myrrh, are helpful for pain and swelling as well as itching. Sitz baths should be limited to one a day while stitches are present. Aloe vera, fresh or gel, and vitamin E are both helpful for healing as is Slippery Elm bark.

## Colostrum

Colostrum is the yellowish liquid that first forms and is expressed from the nipples when breastfeeding begins. It persists for 2 to 3 days before the true breastmilk begins to excrete. It contains a large amount of protein and calories in a small volume that is perfect for the newborn's first few days of feeding. It also contains immune globulins and antibodies for the protection of the newborn. Colostrum has also been found to have a mild laxative effect that helps newborns eliminate the last of the meconium left in their bowels.

## Madonna and Cross Cradle Positions

In the Madonna and cross-cradle positions the infant lays on its side facing the mother. In the football hold, the infant is either on its side or back.

The Madonna, or cradle, position is one in which the head, neck and upper back of the infant are supported by the forearm on the same side as the breast being fed. The opposite hand supports the breast if needed.

The cross-cradle is one in which the mother's hand supports the back of the infant's head and the forearm runs down the infant's back, supporting it to feed on the breast opposite the arm being used. The hand on the same side of the breast being fed supports the breast if needed. In all positions, the use of pillows and other support can be crucial to achieving a comfortable position and good latch.

## Football Hold and Side-Lying Positions

The football hold is one in which the infant is nestled at the mother's side with the forearm supporting the back and head to hold it to the breast. The opposite hand supports the breast if needed. A side-lying position is excellent for mothers recovering from abdominal surgery such as caesarian section. It is also useful if the infant is sleeping with the mother since the mother is not required to sit up or rearrange the bedding in order to feed. In fact, in this position, the mother can still sleep while nursing and the infant will be comfortable and safe once feeding on that side is complete. The infant and mother lie facing each other with the infant's mouth at the level of the lower nipple. In all positions, the use of pillows and other support can be crucial to achieving a comfortable position and good latch.

### Proper Latch

A proper latch in breastfeeding virtually eliminates all discomfort and breast pain that can occur when breastfeeding. In a proper latch, the infant begins with a wide open mouth and latches on with an asymmetrical latch. The areola is drawn into the lower portion of the mouth. If the latch is poor, pain and discomfort will result. Eventually, the nipples will crack and possibly bleed, leading to the inability to breastfeed until the nipples heal. If this occurs before breastfeeding is well-established, the mother's intentions to continue to breastfeed may fade, especially if she lacks a support and education network to encourage her to continue and to educate and assist her in attaining proper positioning.

### Maternal Hydration, Maternal Nutrition, and Maternal Rest

As far as is known, human mothers can product unlimited quantities of breastmilk as long as demand is made and answered. This allows a mother to adequately feed multiple infants or an infant and an older baby. Exclusive breastfeeding on demand with no supplementation will ensure an adequate milk supply. If the newborn gains weight and grows at an expected rate, he or she is taking adequate nourishment. It is a fallacy that dehydration, poor nutrition, and lack of rest in the mother will decrease milk production unless she is profoundly malnourished. Few, if any, herbal galactogogues actually increase the quantity of milk. However, it is important for the mother to maintain her health by eating properly, drinking as needed, and obtaining sufficient rest as much as possible.

### Breast Engorgement

Engorgement is a condition where the breast is excessively full. The breast may feel warm or hot, it may have a shiny appearance, and it will feel tight and hard to the touch. Engorgement typically occurs when feedings are not given often enough. The best relief is breastfeeding the baby until the baby stops nursing and ejects the nipple. This is a helpful treatment for blocked ducts as well. If the baby cannot latch onto the breast due to its fullness, ice packs, heat, or manual expression can soften the breast enough to allow latch on to occur. Some homeopathic remedies include Arnica, Bryonia, Phytolacca, and Belladonna. Echinacea is thought the help prevent the progression of engorgement to mastitis. Comfrey leaf compresses or raw cabbage leaves on the breasts also help relieve engorgement.

### Letdown Reflex and Expressing Breastmilk

The letdown reflex is the action of oxytocin on the breast tissue that results in breastmilk flowing into the infant's mouth. It is stimulated by the infant sucking at the nipple but the hormonal response can also be caused by hearing an infant cry. When it is not possible to breastfeed the infant, breastmilk should be expressed to keep production up. The milk can be expressed manually into a container held below the nipple. The mother places her thumb on top of the breast to be expressed where the areola and the breast tissue meet. The forefinger is placed on top in the same position. The fingers draw the areola back into the chest wall while gently compressing the nipple between them. Milk should eject. A mechanical breast pump attempts to mimic a newborn's sucking mechanism to pull milk out of the breast.

### Newborn Reflexes

Proprioceptive reflexes include the gross motor reflexes such as the Moro reflex. It is symmetrical and can be elicited for the first 2 months. Asymmetry can be caused by fracture of the clavicle or humerus, or brachial plexus palsy. Reflex absence may be due to brain damage or immaturity. Intellectual disability can cause the reflex to persist past 4 months.

Exteroceptive reflexes include rooting, grasping, plantar, anal wink, eye reflexes, stepping, and superficial abdominal reflexes. They can be elicited when the infant is in the alert state. Asymmetry, accentuation, or absence of any of these reflexes should be noted and the infant referred to a pediatrician. Many abnormities in these reflexes can be caused by prematurity or some form of brain damage. Parents should be instructed in these reflexes to reassure them of their infant's normality and to observe for problems.

# The Postpartum Period

## Maternal Recovery

The mother requires 10 full days of absolute rest. She should sleep and eat whenever her body tells her she must. She should not become stressed as that will release adrenaline which interferes with the oxytocin release needed for uterine involution. The mother should also be encouraged to walk several times daily, even if the distance is short to stimulate circulation and prevent thrombophlebitis. A jug of water should be at hand at all times to replenish liquids lost by nursing. Her room should be comfortably warm with any baby or personal needs close by. She may need help with a shower. The mother should be relaxed and happy; if she is not, the reason must be found and corrected. The mother should be allowed to talk to you about the birth if she wishes. Remain receptive.

## Postpartum Care After Placental Abruption

If the fetus is alive and delivered there is a high likelihood of hypoxia and need for care in a neonatal intensive care unit, although this is not a certainty. The mother and her partner must be in complete communication with the medical team and the midwife at all times. The partner may require another family member for support if the mother is in emergency surgery or if her health deteriorates suddenly. With a live birth in which the newborn must be in NICU it is helpful to take a photograph for the mother and arrange a parental visit to the newborn as soon as possible. The mother should be encouraged to help care for the baby. If the baby arrives in good health care of the newborn is normal. In fetal demise, counseling and support will be needed for the mother and family. Maternal postpartum complications include DIC, postpartum hemorrhage, renal failure, and pituitary necrosis.

## Day One to Day Two Postpartum Visit

In general, this visit is to assess the mother's emotional well-being and her relationship with the new baby. The environment of the home should be assessed for cleanliness and order, and for availability of food and drink. The room the mother and baby are in should be warm and all baby items easily accessed by the mother. The mother may require assistance for a shower. The following physical assessments are made:

- For the mother
    - Nipples: soreness, cracking - Uterus: normal involution - Lochia: color, odor, and volume
    - Perineum: swelling, especially if tearing or suturing occurred. Assess for cystocele and rectocele at this time. Check for infection of any stitches, and for tenderness
    - Record temperature, pulse, and blood pressure
- For the baby:
    - Cord stump - Skin color: check for jaundice
    - Skin consistency: for dehydration
    - Elimination pattern: check for meconium passing and urination - Feeding pattern and behavior: check for lethargy and high-pitched crying
    - Anything unusual

### Maternal Abnormalities on the Day One Postpartum Visit

Nipples: sore or cracked nipples require assessment of the breastfeeding position and latch. Vitamin E application to the nipple between feedings and giving the baby the less affected breast first will alleviate the problem.

Perineum: remaining swelling may be treated with alternating hold and cold compresses. The perineum should be rinsed twice a day with water and Betadine. Increased swelling may indicate a hematoma. Cystocele and rectocele can be managed with the "elevator exercise". If infection is observed, a physician referral is needed. Tenderness without other symptoms can be managed with sitz baths. If a bowel movement has not yet occurred, recommend fiber rich foods.

Temperature, pulse, blood pressure: Elevated temperature and pulse may indicate dehydration, systemic urinary tract infection, or uterine infection. Elevated blood pressure, especially if also elevated during or right after labor may indicate preeclampsia.

### Day Three to Day Four Postpartum Visit

By this time, breastmilk may have come in and the parents may be extremely tired. The parents' support system should be fully activated. The following physical assessments are performed:

- Mother
  - Breasts: engorgement, cracked nipples
  - Uterus, perineum: lochia color, odor, volume; uterine enlargement, tenderness, perineal cystocele or rectocele
  - Temperature
- Baby
  - Cord stump: cord clamp removal or removal of cord plus placenta in a lotus birth
  - Skin for jaundice
  - Dehydration
  - Behavior, feeding, crying
  - Mother's relationship to breastfeeding: make certain the baby is not being placed on a schedule
  - Sleeping arrangements: co-sleeping or sleeping in separate bed but in the same room.

### One to Two Week Visit

By this visit the mother may be substantially on her own as her partner returns to work and her other support systems return to their routines. Increased lochia flow or a change from a pinkish color back to red indicates overwork. Help is still needed and must be obtained. The mother should be assessed for postpartum blues or postpartum depression. Any perineal repair should be closed. If not overworked, the mother's lochia flow should be less. Breastfeeding should be established. Any cystocele or rectocele should be decreasing if the recommended exercises are being followed. Sexual activity should not be resumed until the lochia has stopped flowing, especially if the mother has stitches. If later the mother reports sensations of pressure in her vagina, extreme fatigue, continued bleeding, or exhaustion, the midwife should arrange for an immediate visit to check the healing process again.

### Six to Eight Week Visit

One reason for this checkup is to make certain sexual activity can now be undertaken. Breastfeeding can cause vaginal dryness and lubrication is important. This is also the time to check the perineum for tenderness and sensitivity if stitches were needed. Emotional well-being is assessed and an earlier visit may be required if the mother calls with feelings of depression or emotional problems. This is often the last visit. The following assessments are performed:

- Uterus: for any continuing enlargement
- Cervix: for firmness and position, perform Pap smear
- Internal muscle tone: exercises must be continued if tone has not returned
- Lacerations or episiotomy: for healing
- Abdominal muscle tone: check for gaping at the juncture of the abdominal muscles from umbilicus to pubis
- Breasts: tenderness or lumps
- Hemoglobin and hematocrit: In case of exhaustion or if hemorrhage occurred during birth
- Diet
- Adjustment to parenting

## Postpartum History

The postpartum history is the perception the mother has of the birth. While taking this history, questions may arise, misperceptions may come to light, and other information validated. The history also includes the assessments made at each postpartum visit: nutritional habits, bladder and bowel function, pain, discomfort, lochia flow, and activity. You must also ask about the feeding method, behavior and sleep cycles of the baby. During the early postpartum period, if the mother is in a hospital, you are expected to ensure the standing orders for first day postpartum in that facility are appropriate for the mother and that they are being carried out.

## Normal Uterus, Lochia and Perineum

The uterus is below the mother's umbilicus and feels firm, not tender. Massage it to remove any clots and place the mother upright briefly before checking the flow of lochia. At this time lochia rubra, or red-brown flow, appears like a heavy period. The odor is fleshy and similar to menstrual blood. The perineum should no longer be swollen. If swelling is apparent, alternating warm and cool compresses and rinsing the perineum twice a day with warm water and Betadine may help decrease swelling. If the swelling is increased and pain is evident, a hematoma may be indicated. At this time, the vaginal canal is checked for hematoma, cystocele and rectocele. Areas with stitches are pulling together and are clean and dry with no sign of infection. Ask mother about pain with urination and whether a bowel movement has yet occurred.

## Lochia

Lochia is uterine discharge that occurs during the postpartum period. It has different shades of color depending on how much time has passed since the birth:

- lochia rubra is red and contains blood. It begins immediately after delivery and lasts two or three days
- Lochia serosa is more pink than red. It persists for seven to eight days and transitions to lochia alba, which is a light pink, yellow or white color
- Lochia alba begins around the tenth day postpartum and persists for two to four weeks

Over the time from immediate postpartum to six or eight weeks, the flow should decrease and the color change from red to pale pink, yellow, or white. Sudden recurrence of bright red vaginal bleeding is abnormal and must be assessed. It may be caused by overwork, uterine atony, or retained placental or membrane products.

## Postpartum Condition of the Uterus, Ovaries, and Cervix

Within the first 24 to 48 hours, the uterus should be just below the umbilicus but still palpable. It should be firm and non-tender. A quick massage and sitting the mother up will help remove any lingering clots. By three to six weeks, the uterus should no longer be palpable abdominally. Also by this time, the cervix should be closed, firm, and positioned high in the vaginal vault. If the mother is breastfeeding, the tone and position may not yet have returned to normal.

If the uterus is still enlarged, there may still be bleeding. Rest, breastfeeding on demand, and good nutritional intake will help recovery. Involuting tea or tincture of black haw and shepherd's purse may also be of value.

The parents should be reminded that ovulation can occur soon after birth and that exclusive breastfeeding is not an effective form of birth control.

## Postpartum Condition of the Vulva, Vagina, Perineum, and Anus

By 24 hours after birth, most swelling of the perineum should be gone unless excessive tissue trauma, tearing, or suturing occurred. Cystocele, rectocele, hemorrhoids, and hematoma can all form after birth due to lacerations or laceration repair. The mother can apply aloe vera gel to stitches that are not healing. Warm water should be poured over the perineum whenever the mother urinates and if she fears her stitches will tear with a bowel movement, she can apply counterpressure with a folded tissue. Constipation is common due to the amount of time since the mother last ate prior to birth. Eating fiber rich foods and remaining hydrated will go a long way toward alleviating this. Scar tissue in the perineum at six weeks can be softened with evening primrose oil.

## Adverse Factors Affecting Breastfeeding

There are medical reasons for supplementing breastfeeding. Supplementation is acceptable if not required in:

- infants whose mothers are extremely ill immediately after birth
- infants who are premature or of very low birth weight
- infants with hypoglycemia that does not improve with breastfeeding
- infants with dehydration or inborn errors of metabolism
- infants whose mothers are taking medication that is passed through breastmilk and is harmful to the infant

The working mother can find it difficult to maintain breastmilk volume after returning to work. She must find a way to express milk during her time at work in such a way that her milk does not diminish due to lack of breastfeeding. The workplace may not be conducive to milk expression or storage.

## Contraceptive Effect of Breastfeeding

When a mother is breastfeeding it is thought that gonadotrophin release is inhibited, especially luteinizing hormone (LH) which then inhibits ovulation. The start of ovulation in a breastfeeding mother varies depending upon the breastfeeding pattern she follows. The return of ovulation depends on nursing frequency, intensity, and duration including night feedings and the advent of solid food. The Lactation Amenorrhea Method (LAM) combines the lack of menstruation experienced after birth with full time breastfeeding to act as a form of family planning during the first six months postpartum. In other words, as long as the mother is not yet menstruating and is exclusively breastfeeding an infant that is 6 months old or younger, there is only a 2% chance that she will become pregnant. Once the infant is older than 6 months, the chances of pregnancy begin to increase.

## Post-Partum Contraception Issues

Many common contraceptive methods are not suitable for a nursing mother.

- IUD can cause chronic bleeding and low grade infection
- Basal body temperature and cervical mucus may not stabilize for some time after the birth and during nursing
- Estrogen/progesterone birth control pills can cause milk production to slow or stop while progesterone-only mini-pills are not as effective for birth control
- Norplant and Depo-Provera can cause heavy bleeding and may delay the start of menstruation when stopped

Barrier methods have the fewest side effects and are most effective for post-partum couples. These include condoms, diaphragms, and cervical caps. Some couples dislike the implied separation of barrier devices and may have the urge to conceive again, albeit subconsciously, and be less than diligent with the device. The couple must consider these issues and come to terms with them prior to resuming intimacy.

## Postpartum Uterine Infection

Signs and symptoms include general malaise, pain, elevated temperature, and lochia with a foul odor. Endometritis, in particular, typically presents with a fever of up to 104 degrees F, chills, tachycardia, pelvic pain during bimanual exam, lateral uterine tenderness, elevation of the white blood count, and subinvolution.

The interpretation of laboratory culture and sensitivity reports as well as treatment should be discussed with the consulting physician. Broad spectrum antibiotics such as the cephalosporins, extended spectrum penicillin, and penicillin with a beta lactimase inhibitor are commonly used. Metronidazole is contraindicated in a breastfeeding mother. Echinacea root has also been used to good effect as a tincture and infusion. Oral antibiotic therapy will suffice unless the infection is severe enough to warrant IV therapy in a hospital facility. If the infection spreads, salpingitis, peritonitis, septic thrombophlebitis, and necrotizing fasciitis may result.

## Postpartum Urinary Tract Infection

A urinary tract infection can be difficult to diagnose in the immediate postpartum since many signs and symptoms are shared by other conditions. If urinary catheterization or vaginal trauma has occurred, there is an increased risk of infection. Symptoms include dysuria, urinary frequency and urgency, and less typically, lower back pain. If the infection progresses to pyelonephritis, flank pain, CVA tenderness, and low grade fever with spiking may occur. A clean-catch urine culture must show an overabundance of a single bacterial type to definitively diagnose the infection.

## Postpartum Infection

Known in earlier times as childbed fever, puerperal (postpartum) infection is caused by introduction of bacteria into the lower genital tract. This can occur:

- during prolonged rupture of the membranes or prolonged labor
- when many vaginal exams are performed during labor
- when aseptic technique is not scrupulously followed
- during or after extensive tissue damage

- during intrauterine manipulation
- with previous untreated disease or infection of the reproductive tract
- with hemorrhage, retention of placental fragments, or poor perineal care

Bacteria involved in this type of infection can be opportunistic pathogens such as those that normally live in the bowel, lower genital tract, or in the nasopharynx. Others are introduced through contaminated hands, gloves, or equipment. These pathogens include *Staphylococcus aureus*, *Gardnerella vaginalis*, *Streptococcus* sp., *E. coli*, *Klebsiella*, *Proteus*, and others.

### Postpartum Infection of a Vaginal Tear or Incision

Postpartum teaching is aimed at preventing such infection. The mother is instructed in care of the postpartum perineum. However, infection may still occur, if only through a moment of carelessness. The tissues in this area may be infected by bacteria from the bowel or from the lower reproductive tract. Infection in a vaginal tear or incision is characterized by redness, tenderness, heat to the touch, and possibly exuding pus or other purulent matter. If it is severe enough, the infection may also cause fever. Treatment with antibiotic cream, oral antibiotics, or IV antibiotics may be used. Warm or cold compresses and oral analgesics can help relieve pain and swelling. Careful cleaning of the area on a regular basis without reopening the wound facilitates healing.

### Post Partum Depression

One in five mothers develop depression or anxiety up to a year after the birth of a baby. Half show at least two signs of clinical depression including:

- loss of interest or pleasure in life
- low energy
- sleep problems
- increased crying or tearfulness
- feelings of worthlessness, hopelessness, guilt, restlessness, irritability or anxiety
- sudden weight loss or gain
- thoughts about self-harm
- worry about hurting the baby

These feelings are caused by hormonal shifts and maternal emotions regarding the baby, the birth experience and the maternal role. Depression may not begin until a baby is weaned and menses returns. A woman with a personal or family history of depression or bipolar illness, or other issues in her life may be more prone to developing post partum depression. You should immediately refer her to the appropriate health care professional if you observe these symptoms.

## PTSD

Many women who have a traumatic birthing experience can overcome any trauma that may have occurred during the birth such as the effects of pain, the experience of an operative birth rather than a natural one, or a suboptimal emotional experience because of disrespectful or indifferent treatment by staff. Others may not be able to overcome these experiences and suffer flashbacks and nightmares along with other issues related to PTSD. Unlike postpartum depression it is not physiologically based, but directly linked to the trauma, fear, and stress of childbirth. At this time, there is no standard treatment for this issue although it has been thought that a brief intervention in which the immediate symptoms of obstetric distress are treated. You can assist by encouraging the mother to talk about her experiences and fears and by reassuring the mother that nightmares can simply be a way to express fear and anxiety.

### Postpartum Psychosis

This is a condition requiring urgent referral for mental health treatment.

Extremely rare but more serious than postpartum depression, postpartum psychosis is characterized by suicidal or infanticidal behaviors as well as delusions. The mother may have manic or depressive episodes. She may suffer from confusion or disorientation, agitation, mood swings, and fear. She may refuse to eat. Onset is rapid, typically within the first week postpartum but rarely before the third day although symptoms may not appear for up to three months. While most suffering from this disorder may be experiencing mental illness for the first time, women with bipolar disorder seem to be at higher risk. It is thought to be caused by biochemical imbalance rather than stress. Medication is usually required for treatment and continued management. It is imperative that this disorder is recognized and treatment administered as early as possible. Although this is a rare condition, it can have extremely serious consequences.

### Late Postpartum Hemorrhage

Late postpartum hemorrhage is defined as profuse bleeding anytime from 24 hours postpartum up to 6 weeks. Commonly it will occur one to two weeks postpartum. Symptoms include bleeding that soaks one sanitary pad in an hour, bleeding is bright red, and blood clots are larger than a golf ball. At its most severe, shock can result. Typically, late postpartum hemorrhage is caused by retained remnants of the placenta or membranes in the uterus or a uterus that does not contract sufficiently due to infection or other conditions. Treatment includes oxytocic medications, removal of any placental or membrane fragments, rest, hydration, and a blood transfusion if needed.

### Thrombophlebitis

Thrombophlebitis is an inflammation of a leg vein. Those with varicose veins are at higher risk than those without.

Superficial thrombophlebitis presents with leg pain, heat, tenderness and redness at the inflamed area. Confirmation of superficial thrombophlebitis can be done by checking for Homan's sign. Thrombophlebitis is superficial if there is pain in the mother's calf when the affected leg is straight and the foot flexed.

Deep thrombophlebitis is indicated if there is a high fever, severe pain, edema and tenderness along the entire leg.

For either problem, the mother should be on bed rest with her leg elevated. Her leg should not be manipulated in any way. If a clot becomes dislodged from her leg and lodges in the lungs, pulmonary edema may result; oxygen must be administered and emergency services notified.

### Physiological and Pathological Jaundice

Physiological jaundice is a non-threatening condition caused by the release of bilirubin during the breakdown of excess red cells in newborn circulation. Bilirubin gives a characteristic yellow tinge to the skin and is seen by the second or third day of life. Other types of physiological jaundice are:

- breast milk jaundice: a hormone in the breast milk interferes with the newborn's ability to eliminate bilirubin
- ABO incompatibility: Maternal Type O blood transfers to a baby with blood-type A or B. Maternal red cell breakdown creates excess bilirubin

Pathological jaundice may be caused by:

- liver disease
- an obstructed bile duct
- infection
- Rh hemolytic disease

Unlike physiological jaundice, pathological jaundice usually:

- presents within the first 24 hours of life
- Bilirubin levels are much higher
- If bilirubin levels are not decreased quickly, kernicterus can result.

Another name for jaundice is hyperbilirubinemia. Any jaundice on the first day should be referred to the pediatrician.

**Review Video: Jaundice/Icterus**
Visit mometrix.com/academy and enter code: 339680

## Circumcision

Circumcision has become a controversial procedure. Education regarding the procedure and its aftermath is essential to make an informed decision for the male infant. In some cultures circumcision is part of religious or family tradition. There is also some evidence that a circumcised penis is more easily cleaned, reducing the incidence of urinary tract infections, cancer and sexually transmitted diseases. However, these potential medical benefits are not significant enough to advocate the procedure for all male infants. If it is to be performed, the American Academy of Pediatrics recommends analgesia via a dorsal nerve block or anesthetic cream prior to surgery. If the decision is made not to circumcise, the parents must be educated in the appearance, development and care of an uncircumcised penis.

## Care of a Circumcised Penis

During the first 24 hours after the circumcision the glans of the penis will appear red and the remaining foreskin may be somewhat edematous. There may be some drainage as well. After one to two days the redness will start to fade and healing will take about a week. The initial dressing of gauze and Vaseline should be left in place for 24 hours unless it becomes soiled, then a fresh gauze and Vaseline dressing should be placed around the penis each time the diaper is changed. Good hand washing will prevent infection. Any redness, swelling, fever over 101 degrees, lethargy, refusal to nurse, pustular drainage, or lack of voiding should be reported to the midwife who did the circumcision or to the pediatrician as the wound is infected. Alcohol and soap should not be used to clean the glans as this is drying and irritating. Once the circumcision is healed and the umbilical stump has fallen off, the infant may have a tub bath.

## Care of an Uncircumcised Penis

The foreskin of an uncircumcised penis on a newborn should never be pulled back. The foreskin will eventually loosen but this may be months or years away. The penis should be cleaned the same as the rest of the baby. Once the foreskin has separated from the penis, it can be gently pulled back periodically and cleaned of the smegma that sometimes accumulates at the tip. Once the child is old enough to bathe himself, he must be taught to do this as well.

## Non-Allopathic Treatments for Thrush on the Nipples

The nipples should be dried after nursing and kept as dry as possible between nursing sessions. Good hygiene is essential for keeping thrush from spreading once it starts. If the infant has oral thrush, it can easily be passed to the mother where thrush forms on the nipples. Yogurt or acidophilus solution has been used to good effect. The infant can suck on a finger with yogurt and yogurt can be smeared on the nipples. It should be washed off before nursing. Another remedy is to discourage thrush from the nipples by bathing them in a vinegar solution of 1 tablespoon of vinegar in 8 ounces of water after nursing. If these remedies do not give relief, the mother should be referred to a physician. Nystatin is a common treatment option.

## Sore Nipples in a Breastfeeding Mother

Sore nipples that are not caused by thrush or another condition can be caused by a poor latch and infrequent nursing (causing the infant to suck extremely aggressively). Ice can be applied to the nipple before nursing to create an analgesic effect and bring out nipples. Comfrey root ointment can soften nipples and speed healing. Yarrow leaf, poultices or ointment can relieve pain and increase the speed of healing. Vitamin E or Aloe vera applied to the nipple can also be beneficial. To prevent sore nipples, Lanolin or expressed milk can be applied to the nipples after each feeding. The nipples should also be exposed to the air for a period of time each day and allowed to air dry before the bra and shirt are refastened. Different nursing positions may also help alleviate some of the problem.

## Mastitis

Mastitis is an infection of the breast. Breast injury or a pathogen that has invaded the tissue can cause mastitis. Engorgement, a blocked milk duct, or cracked nipples can all contribute to the risk of mastitis. Mastitis can be prevented by feeding early and often to emptiness, maintaining good hygiene, and ensuring proper positioning and latch.

Signs and symptoms of mastitis are:

- rapid onset of fever
- increased pulse
- painful, hard area of the breast
- chills
- general malaise

An abscess may develop if the mastitis is not treated. A supportive bra that does not constrict the breast tissue, as an underwire bra tends to do, should be worn. Warm compresses to the affected area will give comfort. Rest, increased fluids, and gentle massage while breastfeeding encourage milk flow and prevents the infection from progressing. Antibiotic therapy will treat any pathogenic agent implicated in the infection. Poke root, Propolis, elder root, and Echinacea root have all been used as remedies as well.

# Well-Baby Care

## Well-Baby Care

The parents are expected to be solely responsible for the infant once the immediate postpartum time has passed. Often, within a week, friends and family who gathered to help with the birth are no longer available. However, the parents are just beginning to realize the reality of life with a newborn, even if this is not a first child. There are still many skills to be learned at a time when rest is at a premium. Assistance from a professional who can educate them and watch them practice these skills is invaluable. The midwife, who has become especially well known and accepted by the parents, will be in a position to immediately answer any questions the parents have in a way that helps them most. Additionally, the midwife is able to watch the infant while it is still adapting to extra-uterine life. He or she may be able to observe conditions or diseases that escape the notice of the parents.

## Newborn Vital Statistics

Temperature: 36.5 - 37.5 C (97.7 – 99.5 F) at birth.

The flexed posture of the newborn helps maintain body temperature. Unstable temperature may indicate infection.

Heart rate: 120 – 160 beats per minute.

There are fluctuations with respiration and activity.

Respiration: 30 -60 breaths per minute.

The newborn is an obligatory nose breather and has periods of apnea for 10 – 15 seconds. There should be no nasal flaring, grunting, sternal or subcostal recession during respiration.

Head circumference: 31 – 38 cm occipital/frontal circumference.

Length: average 19 ¾ inches in the United States and shows fairly steady growth over the first year, adding half again the original newborn length.

Appropriate weight gain: one ounce a day for the first three months.

Initially the newborn may lose up to 10% of the original weight but will gain it back within 2 weeks, a little longer for breastfed babies. Within the first year the weight triples.

## Newborn Sensory Capabilities

The sensory capabilities for a term newborn are:

- ability to visually fix and track objects.
- a strong preference for stripes or patterns, and black, white, and strong colors.
- At two weeks an infant can mimic human facial expressions.
- Discrimination of taste and odor, preferring its own mother's scent and the taste of sweet liquids.
- Localization of sound and discrimination between sounds, showing a preference for human voices over synthesized sounds and picking out its mother's voice from others.
- By one month this preference evolves into preferring sound patterns similar to speech.

Many of the exteroceptive reflexes are related to touch. These reflexes are often survival mechanisms meant to help the infant obtain nutrients and remain safe from danger. Infants also enjoy being touched, especially skin to skin contact.

## Denver II Developmental Screening Test

Of the developmental screening tests available, the Denver II is the most accurate in early infanthood. It compares the infant's skills with the skill sets of a composite group of 2000 infants of the same age. It does not measure intelligence or motor skills so much as it identifies where an infant lays on a continuum of developmental issues. Typically, if an infant is unable to perform a skill that 90% of others in the age group can, that skill is noted for further investigation. However, it is not a diagnostic tool, it is a screen for early identification of children at risk of delayed development. By 8 weeks of age, babies who were born at term should have reached the developmental levels in all four areas tested: personal-social skills, fine motor movements, language, and gross motor capabilities. Any findings of significant difference should be placed in context with other information such as previous developmental patterns and degree of delay.

## Well-Child Visit During Postpartum

The first postpartum visit generally takes place when the infant is 10 to 14 days old and includes reviewing the family history taken to this point. Observe the family interacting with the baby and ask questions about their adjustments, recording the results in the chart. Further history is taken on the newborn, including feeding, bowel, bladder, alertness and crying habits and any concerns noted. The infant's length, weight and head circumference measurements are repeated. The weight should now be back to the birthweight. A physical exam of the baby is performed to ensure continued health and to find any later presenting conditions. If a metabolic screen was taken before the baby was nursing for a full 48 hours, it must be repeated. Offer guidance to the parents and any siblings regarding expectations of the next 6 to 8 weeks when another visit will be scheduled. Finally, tell the parents how to obtain emergency assistance.

## Newborn Sleep-Wake States

The waking states include:

- crying
- much motor activity
- alert
- drowsy

Newborns spend 15% of daytime hours in the alert state. Crying communicates a need to be fed, held, stimulated to suck, or to sleep. Rarely, it is for pain. The sleep states include active (light) sleep and deep sleep. In light sleep, respiratory rates may vary, there are frequent motor movements and the infant can startle easily. In the deep sleep state there are few motor movements and respiration is deep and regular.

Healthy newborns spend up to 60% of their time sleeping, mostly in short naps. Over the first month, many changes take place: the infant begins to spend more time in deep sleep as opposed to light sleep and in the waking states there is an increase in the alert state. There is higher alertness to the world around her even while crying.

## Infant Skin Care and Diaper Choice

Skin care is of most concern in the diaper area. Diaper rash can be prevented by regular diaper changes and thorough cleaning with mild soap and water or a commercial wipe. Barrier creams containing zinc oxide may stop early diaper rash. Otherwise, routine use of oils, powders or lotions is neither needed nor preventative.

Parents must determine the choice of diaper themselves. Some opt for disposable diapers for the convenience. Others oppose them for environmental reasons although commercial diaper services can also pose environmental issues because of bleach use and pollution caused by the delivery trucks. If the parents decide to wash the diapers at home, the diapers must be presoaked in bleach and detergent and then washed twice in hot water to ensure absolute cleanliness. The rinse water should move freely around the diapers so overloading must be avoided.

## Infant Safety in the Home and Car

Infant safety in the home begins from birth. The earliest risks are falling or getting stuck between crib bars. Used equipment and supplies should be inspected for reliability and to insure there are no spaces where the infant's head can be stuck. Crib slats can be no more than two and three-eighths (2 3/8) inches apart. The mattress should fit tightly. The crib should be free of soft bedding and toys that could suffocate the infant.

A child car safety seat is mandated in many states for transporting infants and young children. Newborn infants must be placed facing backwards in the back seat of the car. An extremely small infant may not safely fit into a regular infant car seat so different seats should be tried until a good fit is found.  A car seat that is also a free standing infant carrier is a good safety feature because it can be used in the house decreasing the chance of falling.

## Infant Clothing and Sleep Positioning

An infant is limited in ability to regulate body temperature. If overdressed and overheated the skin color will redden, the infant may become irritable, and the back of the neck will be very warm. Over time, an overly warm infant will appear lethargic. Nonrestrictive clothing near the face will cut cold winds. A good rule to follow is to clothe the infant in as many layers as adults plus one layer. Keep in mind that infants differ in their metabolisms just as adults and will feel the effects of the environment differently.

An infant should be placed on its back to sleep to reduce the risk of SIDS (Sudden Infant Death Syndrome). Since the recommendation for this position was introduced in 1992 the deaths from SIDS have decreased significantly. Soft sleep surfaces, loose bedding, bed sharing, smoking by others in the home, overheating, and preterm birth all appear to increase the incidence of SIDS.

## Physiological Jaundice

Physiological jaundice is common in the newborn, particularly those born prematurely, those with bowel obstructions or infection, or those born at high altitude. If the jaundice is severe enough, the newborn can become lethargic and refuses to breastfeed.  If the jaundice is observable only on the face and upper chest, frequent nursing, at least every two hours, and exposure to sunlight through the window for thirty minutes twice daily should be sufficient to decrease or eliminate the jaundice. If it is more widespread the newborn may need more extensive care under bili-lights with the serum bilirubin checked routinely. The baby should be referred to a pediatrician.

## Newborn Skin and Cord

Newborn skin shows its hydration level. Dry looking skin indicates a dehydrated state. Discuss feeding habits to determine the frequency and volume of feeding. Dehydration should only ensue if the newborn is not feeding adequately or if the newborn spends time in a hot environment in which case some water can be offered to offset any sweating. Inspect the skin for rashes, septic spots, and abrasions. The folds and between the fingers especially need attention. The umbilicus should not show red streaks on the belly near the cord and the cord itself should not be oozing or giving off an odor. Refer any septic spots, red streaks or cord problems to the pediatrician.

## Infant Bathing and Umbilical Care

Infants do not require daily baths. The face, head and the diaper area require cleaning with mild soap whenever they become soiled. The area should be thoroughly dried afterwards. A full bath may be given once the umbilicus has fallen off whenever the parent can commit sufficient time for a relaxed experience. All materials must be at the tub-side and the infant should never be left unattended in the water.

The care of the umbilicus begins immediately after birth. Typical practice is to lightly wipe the umbilicus with alcohol or hydrogen peroxide at each diaper change until the umbilicus falls off. The diaper should not cover the umbilicus. Some references state that the disinfection step is not required. The baby should be observed for oozing at the umbilicus and red streaks on the abdomen near the naval requiring medical attention.

## Newborn Feeding, Urination, and Stool Patterns

Newborn feeding patterns are seen in the eagerness for feeding, coordination of sucking and swallowing, and reflexes during feeding. The newborn clenches its fists, places them under its chin, and wriggle its toes. The sucking is interrupted by rest periods which occur more frequently as the feeding session continues. Most newborns feed 8 to 12 times a day and feeding sessions occur in clusters. Abnormal feeding reflexes can be signs of cerebral damage, a congenital abnormality, or illness.

Note the frequency of stool and urine passage. If no stool is being passed, evaluate for infection, gastrointestinal tract abnormalities, or metabolic errors. Loose stools may indicate sensitivity to glucose. Constipation may be relieved by giving water between feedings. Pale stools may indicate biliary atresia. If little or no urine is being passed, breastfeeding may not be occurring as expected. Very dark urine may be seen in jaundiced newborns.

## Cradle Cap

Cradle cap is an adherent, seborrheic exudate on the infant's scalp. The scalp has flaky, dry skin or thick, oily, yellowish scaling or crusting patches. This is a cosmetic issue. It is not an infection. There is very little agreement on what causes it. Massage the scalp with vegetable or olive oil and a soft brush then shampoo. Another method is application of natural oil to the scalp. Leave it in all night, and shampoo it away the next morning using a soft toothbrush. A very fine tooth comb will help remove the flakes from the hair. When this same condition is noted on the infant's eyebrows, ears, armpits or other folds it is called seborrheic dermatitis. More frequent shampoos, no more than two to three a week, can help clear the rash and prevent it in the future although once gone it rarely presents again prior to adolescence.

## Diaper Rash

Diaper rash occurs when the skin becomes irritated by ammonia in urine and bacteria in stool. Simple diaper rash causes flat, reddened areas without involving the skin folds. Clean with mild soap and water or a commercial wipe. If possible expose the diaper area to the air and ensure frequent diaper changes. Clear the rash using a zinc oxide cream. Alternatively, use bag balm, or aloe vera gel and calendula cream.

If there are erythematous confluent lesions, satellite lesions away from the perineum and anus, and skin fold involvement, it may indicate Candidiasis, a fungal infection caused by *Candida albicans*. Use an antifungal ointment such as nystatin, myconazole or clotrimazole. Hydrocortisone cream and tepid water rinses ease inflammation.

If there is peeling skin, exudates or vesicles, there may be a secondary staph or strep infection. Herpes simplex or histiocytosis can cause a rash. Frequent diaper rashes may be caused by non-hygienic practices.

## Sequelae of Infant Thrush

Oral or perineal thrush, caused by the yeast *Candida albicans,* can develop into more serious forms. Cutaneous candidiasis is a form in which a moist papular or vesicular rash occurs, most commonly on the axillae, umbilicus, or perineum. It is managed by keeping the areas clean and dry, and applying topical antifungals such as nystatin. More seriously, disseminated candidiasis can develop in very low birth weight infants. This is a systemic infection that can cause osteomyelitis, meningitis, endocarditis, pneumonia, and pyelonephritis among other illnesses. Oral flucytosine and intravenous Amphotericin B is required for treatment. These infants often have a history of exposure to systemic steroids, catecholamine infusions, and antibiotics, especially cephalosporins. While this is a situation in which the infant is already receiving medical treatment, awareness is essential for all infants who may become immunocompromised

### *Cause and Treatment of Thrush*

Thrush is caused by the yeast *Candida albicans*. In infant thrush, the infection appears as adherent, white, plaque-like clumps on the tongue, gums and hard palate; or as a red rash on the infant's perineum. The infant may develop thrush from birth, after administration of antibiotics, and from caregivers' hands or feeding equipment. Treat with applications of acidophilus solution three times a day by swab if the thrush is not interfering with nursing. It may take several weeks to subside. Gentian violet may also be used for infant thrush.

Thrush can spread from infant to mother, or it can develop on the breasts if the mother has frequent yeast infections. If only one nipple is infected, prevent spread to the other by careful hygiene. Symptoms include an acute onset of sharp, stabbing pain at the nipple during breastfeeding, burning, or itching. Refer the mother and her baby to a physician for appropriate treatment.

## Colic

Some alternative or homeopathic remedies for colic include crushed fennel or caraway seed tea, light pressure and warm compresses on the infant's belly, massaging clockwise around the umbilicus, or bringing the infant's feet to its ears several times. Chamomilla, Nux Vomica, and Mag Phos have also been used. An adjustment by a chiropractor with infant expertise may help. A simple exercise to try is to place the infant on its back and grasp the feet. The feet and legs are brought up as in a diaper change but the lift is slowly continued until the infant is hanging upside down. The infant may rotate in place. When it seems to be settled in one place, the move is reversed until the infant is on its back again. This exercise can be done daily.

### *Causes and Treatment of Colic*

There does not seem to be any agreement on what causes colic or even if such a condition actually exists. Infant colic is defined as crying and screaming for three to four hours at a time on a daily basis. This behavior peaks between three weeks and three months of age and then gradually subsides. There is no conclusive evidence that colic is caused by the mother's diet. It is possible that products containing cow's milk whey may cause gastrointestinal distress. It is also possible that the infant is very sensitive and is overreacting to its environment. There is no treatment but there are some recommendations for soothing the infant: try to feed the infant, swaddle it, give it a pacifier, talk to it face-to-face with a low, rhythmic voice, using different holds, reduce stimulation in the room, walk with the baby, or take it outside for a walk or car ride.

## Infection in the Newborn

### *Prevention*

Most methods of prevention are common sense. Anyone touching the newborn should have clean hands. Frequent washing with soap and running water is best but if this is unavailable or time is of the essence, alcohol based hand wash solutions can be substituted. Wearing gloves decreases the chance of infection further. Breastfeeding, avoiding breakage of the newborn skin and mucous membranes, and continuing education regarding prevention will help reduce infections. Visitors who have infections or have been exposed to a contagious infection should not be allowed to visit the baby or the mother. If, in spite of all measures, an infection is discovered, early diagnosis and treatment will limit the course of infection and the damage it can cause.

### *Immunity and Modes of Infection*

Newborns lack the immune system to fight off most infections once the innate immunity has been breeched. Infection can be passed from an individual's hands, from within the birth canal, or through the placenta. Preterm newborns are more vulnerable than term newborns because maternal IgG transfer may not yet have occurred.

Innate immunity does not require previous contact with a pathogen and is the first defense against infection. It is conveyed through barriers or chemicals. In humans, this means intact skin and mucous membranes, gastric acid and digestive enzymes. A newborn's skin is easily irritated and broken, and normal flora has not yet colonized the gut and developed the acid and enzymes. Acquired immunity develops as the body is exposed to pathogens. This type of immunity can be passed in some measure by breastfeeding and placental IgG transfer, but a majority of this immunity is developed with time and exposure.

### *Polycythemia*

Polycythemia is defined as a hematocrit greater than 70%, venous. This can occur due to twin-to-twin transfusion in utero or a large placental transfusion. The latter can be caused by holding the newborn below the level of the placenta after birth or by delayed placental clamping. Other risk factors for polycythemia are being small for gestational age, being borne of a diabetic mother, having neonatal hypothyroidism, or having Down syndrome.

Sequelae to polycythemia are hypoglycemia due to the increased number of red cells consuming glucose, apnea, respiratory distress, cardiac failure, or necrotizing enterocolitis. The newborn may also present with jitteriness, irritability, convulsions or a neurological disorder. Treatment is reserved for those exhibiting symptoms. In these cases, a partial exchange using plasma or plasma expanders is performed to reduce the red cell load. Refer a polycythemic newborn to a pediatrician immediately.

### *Diagnosis and Treatment*

Many early signs of infection are difficult to differentiate from other conditions. An infection may be due to prolonged membrane rupture prior to birth, chorioamnionitis, or infection of the amniotic fluid.

It can be diagnosed by abnormal body temperature, urine and stool output. Diagnostic symptoms also include vomiting, lethargy, poor intake of nutrition, hypoxia, acidosis, dehydration, starvation, or central nervous system conditions that require investigation by a neurodevelopmental specialist. A diagnosis of infection can be confirmed by a performing a complete blood count and culturing urine, meconium, nasal, umbilical, pustule, vesicle, amniotic fluid, placental tissue, cord blood or throat secretions. Additional testing includes MRI, CT scan, chest X-rays, or CSF examination through lumbar puncture.

### *Bacterial Infection*

Bacterial infection of the newborn can be differentiated as early onset (birth to 6 days) and late onset (7 days to 3 months). The most common pathogens are Group B beta-hemolytic *Streptococci* and *E. coli.* Other common pathogens are *Staphylococcus aureus* and *Streptococcus epidermidis,* which tend to be nosocomial infections. Early onset bacterial infection can be severe. Symptoms include tachypnea, labored breathing, and poor color. Temperature instability and hypotension may be present. Immediately transport the newborn for emergency treatment.

Late onset bacterial infection usually appears after the newborn has been discharged from daily care by a healthcare worker such as the midwife. Symptoms include lethargy, color changes, lack of sucking, transient apnea, and fever. In these instances, refer the newborn for medical treatment.

### *Congenital Viral and Parasitic Infections*

Congenital viral and parasitic infections are acquired transplacentally and will have different symptoms than infections acquired during birth. Early jaundice, hepatosplenomegaly, petechiae and palpable lymph nodes are some of the signs of this type of infection. The newborn may also be small for gestational age. Additional symptoms of congenital infection can include vesicles, rash, limb or cardiac defects, microcephaly, cataracts, or thrombocytopenia. Visibility of the symptoms or abnormalities depends upon timing of exposure and severity of the infection. The cord blood should be tested for IgM, which signifies a viral infection, and cultured for virus identification. These newborns should be isolated from other newborns and pregnant women until the virus is identified. Some examples of this type of infection are Toxoplasmosis and Varicella (Herpes) Zoster.

## Group B Streptococcus (GBS)

Group B Streptococcus can be found in the vagina or rectum of up to 30% of women, who are at no risk of harm from these bacteria. However, 5% of newborns can become infected during the birthing process. Premature infants are most at risk. Early onset GBS occurs within a few hours of birth. The first symptoms are often lethargy, fever, and difficulty feeding. This can lead to pneumonia, sepsis or meningitis. Late onset GBS occurs a few weeks to a few months after birth and about half the cases are passed from the mother. The symptoms and illnesses are similar to those of early onset GBS but are usually less severe. Even with antibiotic treatment GBS, both early and late onset, can be fatal. Survivors, especially of meningitis, may have long term neurological damage such as seizures and hearing loss.

## RDS

Respiratory Distress Syndrome (RDS) is a medical emergency requiring hospital care. RDS occurs in premature infants who have little or no surfactant in the lungs. RDS is caused in term infants by pneumothorax, aspiration of meconium, pneumonia, and TTN.

A pneumothorax is the rupture of alveoli by air being pushed outward into the interstitial space of the lung. With a large pneumothorax, there are diminished breath sounds on one side, cyanosis, and possibly overdistention of the chest.

Meconium aspiration symptoms include uneven breath sounds, cyanosis, rales, ronchii, and a barrel chest. It can degenerate into persistent pulmonary hypertension.

Pneumonia can be differentiated from meconium aspiration by the presence of hypothermia, color changes, and apnea. Pneumonia can be caused by a variety of pathogens and the intensity of the infection varies.

### Newborn Heart Abnormalities

Cardiac problems in newborns appear similar to respiratory disease and sepsis. Most congenital defects are structural and impact the heart or the major cardiac vessels. Signs include:

- Pallor, transient tachypnea, and central cyanosis.
- Bounding or diminished pulses.
- Variation of pulse intensity from upper to lower extremities.
- Presence of a loud murmur at birth or a week or two later.

Heart disease cyanosis is seen over the whole body differentiating congenital heart abnormalities from peripheral cyanosis of normal newborns. The most common defect is a ventricular septal defect. A large enough defect can degenerate into congestive heart failure. It is not a cyanotic defect and a murmur may not be heard for two or more weeks. Other concerns such as breastfeeding problems, failure to thrive, and tachypnea may point to this condition. Persistent pulmonary hypertension (formerly persistent fetal circulation) is another common defect. Immediately transport these newborns to a hospital.

### Glucose Disorders

The most common glucose disorder is hypoglycemia of the newborn, a reaction to the prenatal environment. It is defined as a blood glucose level of 45 mg/dl or lower. Symptoms include:

- lethargy
- poor feeding
- seizures
- hypothermia
- high-pitched cry
- irregular respirations
- decreased consciousness level

Premature infants, infants of diabetic mothers, sick infants (i.e. septic), and infants with inborn errors of metabolism are at higher risk of neurological damage. Treat these infants promptly. If the blood glucose is close to 45 mg/dl encourage the mother to breastfeed as often as possible and afterwards give the infant water with molasses at a rate of 1 teaspoon of molasses per cup of water. If the glucose level does not rise, medical intervention is required. Hyperglycemia is less severe than hypoglycemia and usually presents in premature and severely growth restricted infants. Generally, no treatment is needed unless there is excess loss of glucose in the urine, causing osmotic diuresis.

### Hypoglycemia

Hypoglycemia refers to abnormally low blood sugar. A blood glucose level should be taken via heel stick. Normal levels for a newborn are 50-60 mg/ml. Levels below 30 mg/ml require immediate intervention.

At risk are infants that are:

- large or small for gestational age
- premature
- postmature
- born of diabetic mothers
- hypoxic or depressed at birth

and they will exhibit:

- apathy
- irregular respiration
- hypothermia
- refusal to nurse
- a high pitched cry

If the level is 45 mg/ml or above, the baby should be nursed as often as possible and given water with molasses every few hours (1 teaspoon per cup). The central nervous system can sustain damage if blood glucose levels are too low. The newborn may require more aggressive treatment.

## Birth Defects

A congenital, or birth, defect is an abnormality in the form, function, or structure of some part of the human body. These defects are categorized as chromosome and gene abnormalities, teratogen-caused abnormalities, abnormalities with multifactor causes, and abnormalities with unknown causes.

In chromosome and gene abnormalities, a defect has occurred in the formation of the gametes or following fertilization; there will either be too little or too much chromosomal material. The clinical presentation depends on the specific abnormality of the chromosomal pattern. Teratogens are agents that increase the incidence of birth defects. The list of known and suspected teratogens continues to grow. Many are prescribed drugs. Others are environmental factors, infectious agents, and maternal disease. Abnormalities with multifactor causes are due to a genetic defect in conjunction with teratogenic effects. Abnormalities with unknown causes are responsible for about 80% of birth defects where no specific agent is known.

### *Atresias*

Three common atresias are esophageal, duodenal, and rectal (accompanied by an imperforate anus).

Esophageal atresia occurs when the canalization of the esophagus is incomplete early in pregnancy and impacts the tracheo-esophageal fistula. Commonly, the upper esophagus ends in a blind upper pouch and the lower esophagus attaches to the trachea. This often happens with polyhydramnios.

Duodenal atresia is the most common site for atresia defects. Persistent vomiting in the first 24 - 36 hours after birth will be the first problem seen. This defect is often seen with others; 30% occur in infants with Down Syndrome. Imperforate anus will be apparent upon close examination of the infant.

Rectal atresia will be signaled by the non-passage of meconium. All infants with these defects should be referred for surgical correction.

### Gastroschisis and Exomphalos

The most common abnormalities of the gastrointestinal system are atresias, gastroschisis, and exomphalos, all requiring surgical correction. Many are diagnosed prenatally via ultrasound.

Gastroschisis is a defect of the abdominal wall with extrusion of the bowel which is not covered by peritoneal sac. There is a high risk of injury and infection.

Exomphalos or oomphalocele is defined by protrusion of the bowel or other viscera through the umbilicus and covered by a sac. Other abnormalities often present in tandem which could delay surgery to enclose the viscera.

In both gastroschisis and exomphalos, cover the herniated contents with clean cellophane wrap or warm sterile saline gauze to protect the organs and to delay fluid and heat loss. Aspirate the stomach contents. Immediately transfer to the hospital.

### Cleft Lip and Cleft Palate

Cleft lip occurs in 1.3 per 1000 births. It may be unilateral or bilateral. Cleft palate is often found in conjunction with cleft lip. The cleft may be in the hard or soft palate, sometimes both. Sometimes the alveolar margins are impacted, sometimes it is the uvula. It is best to examine an infant for cleft palate with a good light rather than palpation. Breastfeeding is possible with unilateral cleft lip but in the case of cleft palate, an orthodontic plate will be necessary. Surgical intervention is not immediately needed. Depending on the physician and the parents, cleft lip may be repaired as early as 2 weeks. Some prefer to wait until 3-4 months in case other defects or concomitant medical conditions come to light. The parents should be referred to a support group to help with education about these defects.

### Malrotation/Volvulus, Meconium Ileus, Hirschsprung's Disease, and Pyloric Stenosis

Malrotation (volvulus) is a defect of the small intestine in which incomplete rotation has occurred causing obstruction. Bilious vomiting and abdominal distention are common. Bile stained vomiting requires emergency medical treatment. Surgical correction is required.

Meconium ileus is seen in cystic fibrosis. The meconium is extremely viscous and often causes an obstruction resulting in abdominal distension and bile-stained vomiting. A definitive diagnosis is made via a sweat test at 4-6 weeks.

Hirschsprung's disease is a defect where the large intestine has a section that is aganglionic; peristalsis is lacking and obstructions, abdominal distension and bile-stained vomit occur. A rectal biopsy confirms the diagnosis and the intestine is usually surgically resected.

Pyloric stenosis is caused by a genetic defect causing hypertrophy of the pyloric sphincter muscles. Typically, the defect is suspected when projectile vomiting occurs at 6 weeks or earlier. It predominates in boys and is corrected with surgery.

### Diaphragmatic Hernia

Diaphragmatic hernia refers to an abnormality of the diaphragm that allows herniation of the abdominal contents into the thoracic cavity. Lung development is impacted more or less depending on the size of the hernia and the gestational age when the hernia occurred. Most of these defects are found on the left side so heart sounds are displaced to the right. If not diagnosed prior to birth, the defect may be suspected if the infant is cyanotic and difficult to resuscitate. The diagnosis is confirmed with chest x-ray. This defect can be found on ultrasound, in which case a hospital birth is highly recommended.

### PIERRE ROBIN SYNDROME

This is a group of three defects of the mouth including hypoplasia of the lower jaw (micrognathia), abnormal attachment of the muscles controlling the tongue, and a central cleft palate. The abnormally attached muscles of the tongue allow it to fall back into the throat and occlude the airway. Feeding is extremely difficult. The infant must breastfed in a prone position and be put to sleep on its stomach to keep the airway clear. Aspiration is highly likely. Equipment for medical intervention must be nearby at all times. A long hospitalization is likely until the mandible has developed enough for the parents to take the infant home.

### CONGENITAL CARDIAC DEFECTS

Congenital cardiac defects are the second most common abnormalities found. About 8 in 1000 live births have congenital heart disease and one-third of those will be symptomatic early in life. Chromosomal and gene defects account for 8% of these abnormalities, 2% are likely caused by teratogens. A single cause of the remaining 80% cannot be specified. Teratogenic damage of cardiac development usually occurs in weeks 3-6 of gestation. More and more cardiac defects are being found by ultrasound but most still depend on observation after birth to discover. Infants present with cardiac defects in two ways: cyanotic and acyanotic congenital heart disease. Cyanotic cardiac defects include (in order of frequency): transposition of the great vessels, pulmonary atresia, Fallot's tetralogy, tricuspid atresia, total anomalous pulmonary venous drainage, and univentricular/complex heart. Acyanotic cardiac defects include (in order of frequency): patent ductus arteriosus, ventricular or atrial septal defects, coarctation of the aorta, and hypoplastic left heart syndrome.

### CHOANAL ATRESIA AND LARYNGEAL STRIDOR

Choanal atresia is a narrowing of the nasal passages with a web of bone or tissue obstructing the nasopharynx. Typified by tachypnea and dyspnea, especially with a bilateral lesion, it is usually diagnosed when the infant is observed breathing by mouth and is unable to breastfeed without becoming cyanotic. Additionally, a nasal catheter cannot be inserted. A unilateral defect may not be noted until the infant feeds and cyanosis and respiratory difficulty occur.

Laryngeal stridor is a noise made on inspiration and becomes worse when crying. This is commonly caused by laryngomalacia from laxity of the laryngeal cartilage. This may take up to 2 years to disappear. If dyspnea or feeding problems also occur, a more severe condition may be present.

### ACYANOTIC CARDIAC DEFECTS

Acyanotic defects include:

- patent ductus arteriosus
- ventricular an atrial septal defects
- coarctation of the aorta
- hypoplastic left heart syndrome

There may be tachypnea, tachycardia, and incipient cyanosis after crying or feeding that will increase greatly once the ductus arteriosus closes with coarctation of the aorta or hypoplastic left heart syndrome. There may be heart murmurs and little or no femoral pulse. Prostaglandin stabilizes and maintains the infant until diagnosis. Coarctation of the aorta can be surgically repaired but hypoplastic left heart syndrome is more difficult to treat and does not have a good long term outcome.

Patent ductus arteriosus, ventricular septal defects and atrial septal defects usually do not require surgery or other medical correction in infancy but monitoring should continue for cardiac problems later in life. While not every heart murmur is a harbinger of heart failure, any report of breathlessness or cyanosis should be referred for medical assistance as soon as possible.

### *Cyanotic Cardiac Defects*

Cyanotic cardiac defects include transposition of the great vessels, pulmonary atresia, Fallot's tetralogy, tricuspid atresia, total anomalous pulmonary venous drainage, and univentricular/complex heart. Infants with cardiac defects have persistent tachycardia, tachypnea and central cyanosis. Administration of 100% oxygen does not improve the condition and, in fact, may be detrimental since it may cause the ductus arteriosus to close. Treatment should be discontinued after 10 minutes with no improvement.

Infants with transposition of the great vessels can be treated with surgery to correct the transposition in later weeks. Infants with pulmonary atresia are stabilized with prostaglandin therapy until surgical correction can be performed. Infants with tricuspid atresia usually have a ventricular septal defect or an atrial septal defect. Sometimes both are present allowing circulation to mix.

Some infants do not show immediate cyanosis but become ill later, such as in the Tetralogy of Fallot. Illness occurs several weeks after birth and degenerates into cyanosis and heart failure.

### *Anencephaly and Microcephaly*

Anencephaly results when the cranial vault does not form. It is visible in ultrasound and very apparent at birth. Most fetuses with the defect do not survive to term but occasionally an infant is liveborn. The parents should be shown the infant, first with the back of the head wrapped and a sensitive, honest explanation of the deformity. They should then be shown the head because, while it is hard for parents to see their infant this way, it is helps them to accept the reality of what they are facing and keeps them from imagining anything worse.

Microcephaly is a feature of fetal alcohol syndrome. It can also be seen as a result of a prenatal infection, such as rubella, or as one of the defects in trisomic syndromes. The occipitofrontal circumference is more than 2 standard deviations below normal for the gestational age. Learning difficulties, cerebral palsy and/or seizures will most likely result.

### *Central Nervous System Defects*

Most central nervous system defects are due to a failure of the neural tube to fuse shut, leading to openings in the covering of the spinal cord, or failure of the cranial vault to develop. Central nervous system defects can be prevented by appropriate supplements of folic acid during preconception and pregnancy. These abnormalities are more often discovered prenatally with today's technology, such as detailed ultrasound screening, and parents may choose to terminate the pregnancy when severe neural tube defects are identified. This has led to fewer infants born with these defects. Central nervous system defects include anencephaly, spina bifida aperta, spina bifida occulta, hydrocephalus, and microcephaly.

### *Polydactyly and Syndactyly*

Polydactyly and syndactyly are both musculoskeletal defects in the structure of the fingers or toes. Polydactyly is defined as extra digits and syndactyly refers to webbing between the digits, possibly complete fusion. The fingers and toes should be carefully counted and separated during the birth examination. Polydactyly may result in one or more fully formed extra digits or there may only be extra tissue attached by a pedicle. Syndactyly usually affects the hands. It can occur independently or as part of a syndrome. Surgical procedures are available for both of these issues. It is common to have family history of these types of defects.

### *Hydrocephalus and Spina Bifida*

Hydrocephalus is caused by a blockage in the circulation and absorption of the CSF in the lateral brain ventricles which swell and compress the brain tissue around them. Characteristics are large tense anterior fontanelle, splayed skull sutures, increased occipitofrontal circumference, "sun-setting" eyes, and irritability or abnormal movements. It can be managed with a ventriculoperitoneal shunt.

Spina bifida aperta is caused by failure of the vertebral column to fuse. The area has no skin covering resulting in a meningocele or myelomeningocele. The lesions may rupture and expose the neural tissue. This often occurs at the lumbosacral area but can be anywhere on the vertebral column. An encephalocele is a myelomeningocele at the base of the skull and may contain brain tissue. At birth cover open lesions with a non-adherent bandage and take care not to damage the sac.

Spina bifida occulta is a minor defect with no spinal cord involvement.

### *Talipes*

Talipes is commonly known as clubfoot. Talipes equinovarus, TEV, is a defect in which the ankle is plantarflexed, or bent downwards, and the front part of the foot turns inwards. This form of talipes is likely to occur along with spina bifida defects. Talipes calcaneovalgus is where the ankle is dorsiflexed, or bent upwards, and the front part of the foot is turned outwards. Both of these types of defects occur most often due to crowded conditions in utero as in multiple pregnancies, oligohydramnios, or a macrosomic fetus. Talipes is more common in males than females and sometimes there is a family history of the condition. Mild forms can be corrected with exercise and manipulation while severe forms may need surgery, splinting, and/or manipulation. Early treatment is highly recommended.

### *Limb Reduction Defects*

There has been no success in finding any singular cause of limb reduction defects. These defects can be due to arrested development, as in the absence of part or all of an appendage, or longitudinal arrest of the limb as in fingers or a hand appearing at the end of a severely foreshortened arm. In the latter case, thalidomide has been identified as a major teratogen causing this issue. Cases of a particular type of defect may be clustered in a geographical area but even then a cause may not be found. Supportive care, not only of the infant, but of the parents, is of the most importance. The infant can be fitted with prostheses and may benefit from corrective surgery. Most will adapt to their defect and to any treatment. Refer parents to support groups where available.

### *Achondoplasia and Osteogenesis Imperfecta*

Achondoplasia describes and infant with a disproportionately large head and short limbs. Cognitive development is not generally affected. Most are new mutations with no previous family history. The infant may develop significant lordosis.

Osteogenesis imperfecta is a defect in collagen production and results in brittle bones. There are four types. Types II through IV lead to multiple fractures of the skull, ribs and long bones in utero or during birth. In either case, the fetus may die. Genetic counseling is advised prior to future pregnancies.

### Developmental Hip Dysplasia

Hip dysplasia occurs most often in breech birth or oligohydramnios and more often in first pregnancies and in female infants. The left hip tends to be the one affected. The hip may be dislocated, easily dislocatable, or have subluxion at the joint. Only an experienced health care worker should perform the examination for this, using either Ortolani's test or Barlow's test. An ultrasound of the hips and a referral to an orthopedic specialist is recommended. Treatment is commonly performed by using a special splint or a harness.

### Genitourinary System Defects

A single umbilical artery in the umbilical cord or abnormal facies associated with Potter's Syndrome may be found at birth. These are usually the first symptoms observed in infants with genitourinary system defects. It should be noted whether urination occurs after birth. Observation should continue for 24 hours; if no urination occurs or urine is constantly dribbling, the infant should be referred to the pediatrician. A constant, dribbling urine stream is indicative of nerve damage as is seen in neural tube defects. A poor urine stream is seen in lower urinary tract obstruction. Abnormalities include ambiguous genitalia, polycystic kidneys, hypospadias, cryptorchidism and posterior urethral valve(s).

### Abnormalities of the Skin

Capillary malformations and capillary hemangiomata are both vascular nevi and are defects in skin development. Capillary malformations affect the dermal capillaries. A common defect of this type is the "stork mark", usually on the back of the neck. These generally fade. A more obvious defect of this type is the port wine stain which affects mostly females. It does not fade but laser treatments and makeup can disguise it. Psychological support will be needed. Capillary hemangiomata arise after a few weeks and are typically red, raised lesions. They are most often seen in premature infants, more likely females. The lesions will increase for a time then regress until they disappear at age 5-6 years. Melanocytic (pigmented) nevi are brown, possibly hairy marks that may be raised or flat and vary in size. Because some of these result in malignancies, they are often surgically removed.

### Cryptorchidism and Ambiguous Genitalia

Cryptorchidism is defined as undescended testes. Impacting male infants, this defect can be unilateral or bilateral with an occurrence rate of 1-2%. At birth the scrotal sac(s) will be empty. If the undescended testes are in the inguinal pouch it is possible to manipulate them into the scrotal pouch where it is likely they will continue to develop normally. If the testes are too high in the inguinal pouch to manipulate, they may be malformed. Regular examinations are advised. If the testis has not descended by 2 years of age, surgery may be needed.

The appearance of ambiguous genitalia can be seen as any of the following: an enlarged clitoris or undescended testes, incompletely separated or poorly differentiated labia, a small hypoplastic penis, bifid scrotum or chordee. There are many causes of ambiguous genitalia. Refer such infants for expert medical assistance in clarification of gender.

### Posterior Urethral Valve(s), Polycystic Kidneys, and Hypospadias

Posterior urethral valve(s) defects affect male infants. Urine is prevented from flowing normally out of the body due to valves occurring in the posterior urethra. This in turn causes bladder distension, back pressure on the ureters and the kidneys, and concluding in hydronephrosis. This abnormality may be diagnosed and treated within the uterus; otherwise early diagnosis and treatment postnatally is urgent although severe renal damage may have already occurred. Surgical and other treatments are available.

Polycystic kidneys can cause birthing problems because the infant's abdomen is larger in circumference than a normal infant. The kidneys are palpable and confirmation is done via ultrasound and radiological exam. The most common outcome is renal failure.

Hypospadias is also a defect of the male genitourinary system. It results in the urethral opening being placed elsewhere on the penis than the tip, as far back as the perineum. This defect is typically associated with chordee. Surgical intervention may be necessary to allow normal urination and sexual function.

### *Trisomy 21 (Down Syndrome)*

Trisomy 21, or Down syndrome, is so-called because the 21st chromosome is tripled. The risk of Down syndrome increases with the age of the mother. The syndrome can be definitively diagnosed with amniocentesis prenatally but the extent of intellectual disability cannot be determined. There are many physical features that may be present in the infant such as widely set, obliquely slanted eyes, a small nose, a rough thick tongue, a small head with flat occiput, broad, squat hands with stubby fingers and incurving small finger, simian crease and generalized hypotonia. Not all features are present in every Down's infant. Do not make a statement based on observations of these features, however suggest the possibility to the parents and gain consent for testing. Down's infants also have higher incidence of cardiac abnormalities, leukemia, and hypothyroidism. Intellectual disability is also present with typical IQs of 40-80. Genetic counseling should be offered for future pregnancy risk.

### *Congenital Hyperplasia and Intersex*

Congenital adrenal hyperplasia is one cause of ambiguous genitalia. The adrenal gland overproduces androgens due to an enzyme deficiency. This problem may not be immediately apparent in male infants. The condition also causes loss of sodium from the body and concomitant imbalances in electrolytes and glucose as well as other blood chemistries.

When internal reproductive organs do not match the appearance of the external reproductive organs it is called intersex. The identification of gender is performed by ultrasound examination of the internal organs but gender assignment is delayed for chromosomal studies, hormone assays, and determination of surgical intervention. It is extremely rare to see true hermaphroditism. Parents experience anxiety, being unable to tell others the gender of their infant nor to choose a name (although androgynous name choices may be made). Most commonly an infant with extremely ambiguous gender is raised as a female.

### *Potter Syndrome, Turner Syndrome, and Klinefelter Syndrome*

Potter syndrome is a fatal condition generally resulting in stillbirth or death soon after birth. It is caused by compressive effects of oligohydramnios either in renal agenesis or severe hypoplasia. Severe asphyxiation at birth is common due to lung hypoplasia. The face is flattened, with low set ears, antimongoloid slant to the eyes with heavy epicanthic folds and a beaked nose.

Turner syndrome, or XO, is a genetic abnormality where only one sex chromosome exists, always an X. The missing chromosome is designated O. The infant is female with a short, webbed neck, edematous feet, and widely spaced nipples, underdeveloped genitalia, and reproductive organs that do not mature. Puberty will not occur, and often is the time diagnosis. Mental development is typically normal but congenital cardiac defects may be present.

Klinefelter syndrome, or XXY, is the presence of an extra female chromosome. It only affects males and is also not typically diagnosed until the absence of puberty.

### *Trisomy 18 and Trisomy 13*

Trisomy 18, in which the 18th chromosome is tripled, presents physically with a small head, a flattened forehead, receding chin, low-set and malformed ears, and often a cleft palate. The sternum is generally short, the fingers may overlap and the feet have the rocker bottom appearance typical of the syndrome. Cardiovascular and gastrointestinal defects are common. These infants rarely live out the first year.

Trisomy 13, also known as Patau syndrome, has a tripled 13th chromosome. These infants are also short-lived, rarely living beyond the age of 3. Physical manifestations are as follows:

- small stature with microcephaly
- limb defects
- midline facial defects such as cleft lip and cleft palate
- brain, renal, and cardiac defects

### Failure to Thrive

Failure to thrive is a condition where the infant cannot obtain, retain, or use enough calories needed to grow and are small when compared to age related norms. Either weight or length are lower than the third percentile or are decreased by more than two major percentiles from one measurement to the next. In the first year of life, failure to thrive is generally due to an organ system issue. Infections, intolerance to milk proteins, chronic illness, problems with the gastrointestinal system, such as chronic diarrhea or cystic fibrosis (which causes a malabsorption disorder), can all cause failure to thrive, as can physical and metabolic disorders. Occasionally, there may be a social factor. It is possible that parents who are worried about an overweight child will limit the infant's nutritional intake. Social issues can contribute to this condition, including poverty. Sadly, it can also be attributed to child abuse.

### Newborn Hemorrhagic Disease

Hemorrhagic Disease of the Newborn (HDN) occurs when there is a deficiency of Vitamin K.

Symptoms of HDN are:

- bruising
- bleeding from the umbilicus, nose, scalp, or puncture sites
- gastrointestinal bleeding

HDN may be implicated by severe jaundice for more than 1 week or persistent jaundice for more than 2 weeks.

HDN occurs in three forms:

- early (0 – 24 hours)
- classic (1 – 7 days)
- late (1-12 months with peak onset before 8 weeks)

Early HDN is rare and impacts infants born to mothers who took warfarin, phenobarbital or phenytoin during pregnancy. Prevention is administration of Vitamin K in the last weeks of pregnancy. Classic HDN strikes infants with birth trauma, postnatal hypoxia, asphyxia, prematurity, antibiotic therapy disrupting normal gut flora, or poor enteral feeding. Late HDN occurs in breastfed infants or those with liver disease and Vitamin K absorption disruption in the bowel, as in cystic fibrosis. Injection of Vitamin K intramuscularly within the first hour of birth is preventative.

## Fetal Alcohol Syndrome

Alcohol has been shown to directly impact fetal development. It is rare that a specific teratogen is discovered and its effect defined so well. If the psychosocial markers for alcohol use are present fetal alcohol syndrome and uterine growth restriction can result. When the infant is born, there are a number of visible physical abnormalities:

- growth-restriction
- low set ears
- small upturned nose
- thin upper lip
- flat facies
- close-set eyes with heavy epicanthic folds
- microcephaly

Some of the features will become more normal looking as the infant grows but the resultant intellectual disability, microcephaly and small body size will still mark the child. The infant may have acute withdrawal symptoms and require therapy. The midwife should counsel and support the parents and refer them to appropriate medical help and social services.

## Child Protective Procedures

Pregnancy and the birth of a child are stressful times for a woman and her partner or family. You are in an excellent position to observe the family dynamic and honestly discuss ways to cope with this stress, in part to decrease the possibility of child abuse. You are also in a position to observe whether a child may need protection because earlier intervention did not prevent the abuse from occurring. It is essential to keep excellent records of any suspected abusive behavior or signs of abuse and any attempted intervention and communication to other professionals or services regarding the family. Abuse includes physical abuse, sexual abuse, emotional abuse, and neglect. You must be fully cognizant of the child protection laws and services in your area.

## Integration of the Infant into the Family

Assisting the integration of the newborn into the family is an important part of aftercare. You should encourage the parent's attachment process as well as help any siblings learn about the new infant. The infant should remain with the mother as much as possible. The infant's name should be used anytime a parent interacts with the infant. Including the father in all discussions, decisions and care of the infant will draw the parents closer together in caring for the newborn and each other. Another point of integration is the education of the parents in feeding, bathing, clothing and diapering the infant. The operative word is "educate": you should not take over from the parents; you should encourage the parents to find the best way to do for themselves. You can also act as gatekeeper, minimizing the visitation of extended family and friends to help the bonding experience between mother and newborn.

## Newborn Metabolic Screening

Every state in the United States requires newborn metabolic screening for congenital hypothyroidism and phenylketonuria. Beyond these two tests, each state may require additional screening tests. You must become familiar with the requirements of the state in which you practice. If the sample is taken before the infant has been feeding for at least 48 hours, the test will be invalid. In this case, a followup screening must be scheduled and collected, either by you or some other agency.

In order to collect the sample appropriately, the instructions with the test must be read and followed. It is important to neither underfill nor overfill the testing areas with blood. The sample should be collected from the lateral underside of the infant's heel and placed on the sample areas according to the instructions for the test.

## Information for Continued Care and Wellness

Your strength is your experience of normal pregnancy and birth. Due to the relationship built between yourself and the mother, you are in the best position to offer referrals for ongoing support and care. As you have been present throughout the pregnancy, you should provide information best suited to each individual mother regarding medical and social services within your mutual community. Not only must you acquire and continue to update medical knowledge to successfully and safely assist in pregnancy and childbirth, you must acquire and update knowledge of the community within which you work and develop contacts within that community for services your clients may need. Prior to birth you ascertained the existence or type of support the mother had during pregnancy and for the birth. After the final postpartum visit, you must determine a strategy and referral list for that mother and her entire family, including the newest member.

# Certified Midwives Practice Test

Want to take this practice test in an online interactive format?
Check out the online resources page, which includes interactive practice questions and much more: **mometrix.com/resources719/midwives**

**1. Upon completion of the vaginal exam, the midwife conducts a digital rectal exam and feels no abnormalities, but the exam elicits bright red bleeding evident on the gloved finger. What is the most likely cause?**

a. Internal hemorrhoid
b. Rectal polyp
c. Anal fissure
d. Rectal carcinoma

**2. At 26 weeks' gestation, a woman complains of blurred vision, increased lethargy, headache, increased thirst, and frequent urination. The initial laboratory assessment should be to assess for**

a. hypertension.
b. hypothyroidism.
c. gestational diabetes.
d. malnutrition.

**3. A pregnant woman is Rh-negative and her partner is Rh-positive. When should the woman initially receive RhoGAM?**

a. At 12 weeks' gestation
b. At 15 to 20 weeks' gestation
c. At 26 to 28 weeks' gestation
d. At onset of labor

**4. A woman who is para 3 and gravida 7 has had**

a. 7 pregnancies with 3 deliveries of live or stillborn fetus after 20 or more weeks.
b. 7 deliveries of live or stillborn fetus after 20 or more weeks and 3 miscarriages.
c. 7 deliveries after 20 or more weeks, which include 3 live births.
d. 7 full-term pregnancies, which include 3 live births.

**5. Which of the following is an indication of lightening?**

a. Decreased frequency of urination
b. Increased shortness of breath
c. Decreased vaginal secretions
d. Increased ankle edema

**6. A woman is 3 months pregnant and her prenatal laboratory screen for rubella shows a titer of 1:7. The midwife should advise the woman that**

a. this is a normal value.
b. she should avoid those with suspected rubella.
c. she should receive the rubella vaccine immediately.
d. the fetus may already be compromised by rubella infection.

**7. A 40-year old woman is in her first trimester and is concerned that her fetus may have Down syndrome. What is the most appropriate initial first trimester screening for Down syndrome?**

a. Ultrasound and quad-screen (alpha fetoprotein, estriol, HCG and inhibin A)
b. Amniocentesis
c. Chorionic villus sampling
d. Ultrasound and pregnancy-associated plasma protein-A (PAPP-A) and human chorionic gonadotropin (hCG) testing

**8. A postpartum mother is experiencing severe cramping afterpains, especially when she breastfeeds her infant. What is the best solution for the mother?**

a. Withhold breastfeeding until afterpains stop.
b. Apply warm compress to abdomen.
c. Take acetaminophen or ibuprofen before breastfeeding.
d. Take an opioid analgesia, such as codeine, before breastfeeding.

**9. A mother brings her term infant (and first child) for an exam 2 weeks after birth. The baby has not regained birth weight, appears listless, has a drawn face, and exhibits poor skin turgor. The mother is breastfeeding. The most appropriate first action is to**

a. question mother about nursing technique and frequency and observe the infant nursing.
b. report the mother to child protective services for neglect.
c. advise the mother to stop breastfeeding and switch to formula.
d. refer mother to a breastfeeding support group.

**10. If a patient's membranes rupture and meconium-stained amniotic fluid is noted, what should be the next step?**

a. Fetal scalp blood sampling
b. Referral for Cesarean section
c. Increased fetal monitoring
d. Ultrasound

**11. When assessing fetal heart rate (FHR) patterns, tachycardia is a heart rate great than**

a. 110 bpm.
b. 120 bpm.
c. 140 bpm.
d. 160 bpm.

**12. A neonate is at 40 weeks' gestation and nursing well but has onset of jaundice at 36 hours. Total serum bilirubin is 12 mg/dL. At this time, treatment should include**

a. continued observation and jaundice assessment.
b. phototherapy.
c. exchange transfusion.
d. discontinuation of breastfeeding.

**13. A woman in labor shows cervical dilation of 2.5 cm and has regular moderate contractions every 15 minutes, lasting 20 seconds. Which stage of labor is the woman experiencing?**

a. Second stage
b. First stage, transition phase
c. First stage, active phase
d. First stage, latent phase

**14. During the initial physical examination, the neonate's chest circumference is 34 cm. What is the expected head circumference?**

a. 32 cm
b. 34 cm
c. 36 cm
d. 38 cm

**15. When conducting an examination of the patient's neck, the correct method for examining the thyroid gland is to palpate the thyroid while standing**

a. in front of patient with the patient's neck extended.
b. in front of patient with the patient's neck flexed.
c. behind the patient with the patient's neck extended.
d. behind the patient with the patient's neck flexed.

**16. On the APGAR scale, what is a good score at 1 minute?**

a. 4
b. 5
c. 8
d. 11

**17. A neonate, 2 days after birth, develops a generalized rash with erythematous papules, vesicles, and some pustules everywhere but on the palms and soles of feet. What is the most likely diagnosis?**

a. Erythema toxicum
b. Neonatal pustular melanosis
c. Cutis marmorata
d. Epidermolysis bullosa

**18. During delivery, shoulder dystocia is evident. The midwife's initial action should be to**

a. apply suprapubic pressure externally over the wedged shoulder.
b. pull the posterior arm out of the birth canal.
c. lift and hyperflex the woman's thighs (McRoberts maneuver).
d. manually rotate the infant's head and upper body.

**19. Ultrasound examination shows a woman has a partial placenta previa with the placenta to the margin of the cervical opening. The mid-wife should**

a. do a vaginal examination with a speculum.
b. do a digital vaginal examination.
c. do a follow-up exam in 2 weeks.
d. refer to specialist.

**20. A neonate who was exposed to maternal herpes simplex virus (HSV). How should the neonate be treated?**

a. No treatment will be effective.
b. Administer IV acyclovir.
c. Administer topical acyclovir.
d. Administer IV immunoglobulin.

**21. When conducting a scalp stimulation test during labor, what is a normal fetal response?**

a. Increased heart rate by 5 bpm for 5 seconds
b. Increased heart rate by 15 bpm for 15 seconds
c. Decreased heart rate by 5 bpm for 5 seconds
d. Decreased heart rate by 15 bpm for 15 seconds

**22. The fundal height is usually at the umbilicus at**

a. 16 weeks of gestation.
b. 18 weeks of gestation.
c. 20 weeks of gestation.
d. 22 weeks of gestation.

**23. During labor, a woman's partner grasps the woman's upper arm tightly and rotates the skin outward, creating a burning sensation, during contractions. This is an example of**

a. abuse.
b. touch relaxation.
c. progressive relaxation.
d. dissociation relaxation.

**24. When assessing a woman's psychosocial changes during pregnancy, the midwife should expect a woman in the first trimester to be especially concerned about**

a. changing body image.
b. miscarriage.
c. sexual relations.
d. congenital defects.

**25. When counseling a pregnant woman in the second trimester about nutrition, the midwife should generally advise the woman carrying a singleton to increase caloric intake by**

a. 300 kilocalories a day.
b. 400 kilocalories a day.
c. 600 kilocalories a day.
d. 800 kilocalories a day.

**26. When assessing fetal position, which designated landmark is used for breech presentations?**

a. Occiput
b. Mentum
c. Acromion process
d. Sacrum

**27. When the midwife is examining the mouth of a neonate and eliciting the reflex for tongue extrusion, which of the following is a normal response for the neonate?**

a. Gagging
b. Pushing tongue out of mouth
c. Pulling tongue into mouth
d. Closing mouth

**28. What is the average weight and length of a neonate?**

a. 2500 to 4000 g and 44 to 55 cm
b. 2000 to 3000 g and 44 to 55 cm
c. 2500 to 4000 g and 35 to 45 cm
d. 2000 to 3000 g and 25 to 45 cm

**29. A neonate's skin shows blue-black discoloration on the buttocks and dorsal area. This is an indication of what?**

a. Mottling
b. Nevus vasculosus (strawberry mark)
c. Mongolian spots
d. Nevus flammeus (port-wine stain)

**30. To elicit the Moro reflex, the midwife should**

a. stroke the infant's palm.
b. stroke the side of the infant's face.
c. make a loud sound or give the infant a gentle jolt.
d. touch the infant's mouth.

**31. A woman exhibits persistent hypertension at 14 weeks' gestation. What is the most likely diagnosis?**

a. Chronic hypertension
b. Preeclampsia
c. Hyperthyroidism
d. Anxiety

**32. Which of the following sexually transmitted diseases markedly increases a woman's risk of having an ectopic pregnancy?**

a. Chlamydia
b. Cytomegalovirus
c. Human papilloma virus
d. Gonorrhea

**33. During the prenatal exam, the midwife estimates the woman's BMI is 32, which classifies her weight as obese. Based on this, the midwife should recommend how much weight gain during pregnancy?**

a. 10 pounds
b. 15 pounds
c. 25-35 pounds
d. None

**34. Which of the following is the best candidate for vaginal birth after Cesarean section (VBAC)?**

a. A woman with one previous Cesarean and a low transverse uterine incision
b. A woman with one previous Cesarean and a T or classic incision
c. A woman with one previous Cesarean and a history of myomectomy
d. A woman with one previous Cesarean who insists on having a vaginal birth at home

**35. A pregnant woman in the second trimester complains of increasing low back pain. Which of the following should the midwife recommend to relieve discomfort?**

a. Hot baths
b. Pelvic-tilt exercise and modified exercise program
c. Applying ice to lower back
d. Acetaminophen

**36. Which of the following places the fetus at risk for asymmetric intrauterine growth restriction (IUGR)?**

a. History of heroin use by mother
b. Severe malnutrition
c. Chronic maternal hypertension
d. Preeclampsia

**37. On day 2 postpartum, a mother reports her lochia remains dark red and has a few dime-sized clots and she is concerned she is bleeding. The midwife should**

a. reassure her that this is normal discharge.
b. request a CBC.
c. refer her for consultation.
d. advise increased oral iron.

**38. A mother develops mastitis and is taking antibiotics but is very uncomfortable. The midwife should advise the mother to**

a. avoid nursing on the affected side.
b. use nipple guards when breastfeeding.
c. massage the breasts in a warm shower.
d. stop breastfeeding because she may infect the infant.

**39. At 4 weeks postpartum, a mother reports that she has begun sleeping excessively and crying, and that she feels out of control and angry toward her infant. The midwife should**

a. discuss postpartum depression and advise the mother to put the child in daycare.
b. discuss postpartum depression and make a referral for a psychiatric consult.
c. advise the patient that these feelings are normal.
d. contact child protective services.

**40. At 3 days postpartum, the mother has developed painfully engorged breasts. The midwife should advise the mother to**

a. use a breast pump to reduce engorgement.
b. apply warm compresses.
c. decrease nursing frequency to every 3 to 4 hours.
d. increase nursing frequency to every 2 to 3 hours.

**41. On examining the neonate, the midwife notes 9 café au lait spots with a diameter greater than 5 mm and freckles on the axilla and inguinal area. The infant should be tested for**

a. neurofibromatosis, type 1.
b. Sturge-Weber syndrome.
c. Addison disease.
d. HIV.

**42. Which of the following grooming products is safe for a pregnant woman to use?**

a. Cleansing preparations with retinoids
b. Hair dye
c. Sunscreen products
d. Permanent waves

**43. The initial response to a woman in suspected preterm labor is to**

a. determine status of the cervix.
b. administer a tocolytic agent.
c. obtain a urine specimen for urinalysis and culture.
d. do an ultrasound.

**44. What is the most common neonatal injury associated with macrosomia?**

a. Brachial plexus injury
b. Shoulder dystocia
c. Hip dysplasia
d. Brain trauma

**45. Which labor and childbirth method encourages women to take an active part in the birthing process and encourages alternatives to hospital birthing?**

a. Bradley
b. Lamaze
c. HypoBirthing
d. Kitzinger

**46. A woman with mild preeclampsia and blood pressure of 150-160/90-100 mm Hg and an immature fetus is usually treated initially with what?**

a. Antihypertensives
b. Magnesium sulfate
c. Bed rest
d. Anticonvulsants

**47. Which of the following procedures can be used to decrease the risk of episiotomy?**

a. Encouraging the woman to hold her breath during second-stage pushing
b. Placing the woman in the lithotomy position
c. Encouraging the woman to respond to her own urge to push
d. Taking measures to speed the second stage

**48. Twenty-five minutes after delivery, there are signs of placental separation and the fundus is firm, but the mother is unable to expel the placenta with bearing down. At this point the best action is probably to**

a. wait for the placenta to expel naturally.
b. apply gentle traction to the cord while applying pressure to the fundus.
c. apply pressure to the fundus.
d. apply moderate traction to the cord.

**49. A woman's membranes have ruptured and fetal heart rate shows bradycardia and moderate nonperiodic decelerations. On digital exam, the midwife feels a loop of prolapsed cord. While awaiting the Cesarean section, the midwife should**

a. remove the gloved finger and administer oxygen.
b. remove the gloved finger, insert a speculum, and reapply pressure to the presenting part.
c. leave the gloved finger in the vagina, push the presenting part upward, and elevate the mother's knees to her chest.
d. leave the gloved finger in the vagina, push the presenting part upward, and apply pressure to the abdomen to change fetal position.

**50. When conducting a prenatal exam, the midwife notes that the woman has rhinorrhea, nasal irritation, and a perforated septum. The midwife should suspect what?**

a. Allergic rhinitis
b. Acute rhinitis
c. Nasal polyps
d. Intranasal drug use

# Answer Key and Explanations

**1. A:** Internal hemorrhoids: Usually not palpable but rectal exam may elicit bright red bleeding. Rectal polyps: Pedunculated or sessile in varying sizes; may be difficult to palpate. Anal fissure: Painful ulceration in anal canal, often with sentinel skin tag posterior to fissure and spastic sphincter. Rectal carcinoma: Polypoid or firm and nodular mass. The rectal exam is usually done after the examination of female genitalia with the woman in lithotomy position to accommodate bimanual palpation. The patient bears down to relax the sphincters.

**2. C:** While these symptoms are fairly nonspecific and may be common to pregnancy, the combination of symptoms, including blurred vision, suggests a possibility of gestational diabetes (which usually occurs during weeks 24 to 28). The initial assessment is generally the 1-hour glucose screening, which requires the patient to ingest 50 g of glucose and have blood drawn one hour later for plasma glucose. If the value exceeds 135 to 140, then the 3-hour glucose tolerance tests is usually conducted with 2 or more abnormal values on the 3-hour test diagnostic of gestational diabetes.

**3. C:** Women who are Rh- with an Rh+ mate receive the serum RhoGAM, containing anti-Rh+ antibodies. These antibodies agglutinate any fetal red blood cells that pass over into the mother's circulatory system and thus prevent the mother from forming antibodies that would attack the infant and sensitize her for future pregnancies.

The mother receives 300 ⍰g RhoGAM (Rhlg, Rh immunoglobulin) intramuscularly at 26 to 28 weeks of pregnancy and again within 72 hours after her delivery. In the case of miscarriage, ectopic, or abortion occurring at 12 weeks or less, the mother receives 50 ⍰g of MICRhoGAM. At 13 weeks or more, the mother receives RhoGAM as for pregnancy.

**4. A:**

| | |
|---|---|
| Gravida | Any pregnancy (including present) regardless of duration/outcome |
| Nulligravida | A woman who has never been pregnant |
| Primigravida | A woman with her first pregnancy |
| Multigravida | A woman in her 2nd pregnancy (or more) |
| Para | Delivery of live or stillborn fetus/neonate after 20 or more weeks' gestation |
| Nullipara | A woman who has not given birth after 20 or more weeks' gestation |
| Primipara | A woman who has given birth, live or stillborn, 1 time after 20 or more weeks' gestation |
| Multipara | A woman who has given birth, live or stillborn, 2 or more times after 20 or more weeks' gestation |
| Grand multipara | A woman who has given birth, live or stillborn, 5 or more times after 20 or more weeks' gestation |

**5. D:** With lightening, as the fetal head engages and moves toward the birth canal, the fundal pressure on the diaphragm lessens, so the mother can breathe more easily; but pressure in the pelvic area increases, causing urinary frequency. The lower abdomen may protrude more than previously. Increased circulatory impairment may cause venous stasis and ankle edema and increased vaginal secretions, as vaginal mucous membranes become congested. Pressure on the nerves may result in leg cramps or increased pelvic and leg pain.

**6. B:** A level greater than or equal to 1:18 indicates immunity while a level less than 1:8 indicates susceptibility to rubella, for which there is no effective treatment. However, the rubella vaccine, which is a live attenuated vaccine, cannot be administered to pregnant women, so the woman should be advised to avoid contact with those with suspected rubella during her pregnancy and should receive the vaccination postpartum as the vaccination at that time poses no risk to the neonate and does not preclude breastfeeding.

**7. D:** First trimester testing for Down syndrome usually involves ultrasound at week 11 and pregnancy-associated plasma protein-A (PAPP-A) and human chorionic gonadotropin (hCG) testing at week 13, although women should be made aware that this test may show false positives. Both amniocentesis (done after 15 weeks) and chorionic villus sampling (done between weeks 9 and 14) are invasive and pose a small risk of miscarriage. The combination of ultrasound during first trimester and quad-screen (alpha fetoprotein, estriol, HCG and inhibin A) during second trimester is more accurate than first trimester testing.

**8. C:** Breastfeeding naturally stimulates release of oxytocin, so nursing may cause afterpains. Analgesic agents such as acetaminophen or ibuprofen, especially an hour before nursing and at bedtime, may relieve discomfort and do not adversely affect the infant. With a first pregnancy, the uterus usually remains contracted after delivery. But with subsequent pregnancies or complications, such as hydramnios or retention of clots or placental tissue, the uterus may alternate between contraction and relaxation, causing severe cramp-like afterpains in the 2-3 days after delivery. Additionally, if the mother receives oxytocin to stimulate contractions, this may increase discomfort.

**9. A:** The mother should be questioned about her nursing technique and frequency and be observed while nursing the child. Since this is her first child, she may need further assistance in nursing properly to ensure the infant receives adequate nutrition. While further tests may be indicated, these signs are indicative of dehydration and poor nutrition, so that should be dealt with first. Since there are no other indications of neglect, referral to child protective services is not appropriate at this time. Switching from breast milk to formula is rarely necessary if the mother receives adequate support and instruction.

**10. C:** While previous standards advised for immediate Cesarean in the context of meconium-stained amniotic fluid, this is no longer advised. Instead, the fetus should be closely monitored for signs of distress and the appropriate team should be present at the birth of the neonate due to risks for respiratory distress secondary to aspiration. These neonates should not be routinely suctioned and/or intubated unless they are nonvigorous and do not respond to noninvasive interventions.

**11. D:** FHR patterns are evaluated based on a baseline rate (rate for 10 minutes between contractions), usually 110-160 bpm. Bradycardia is a rate less than 120 bmp; and tachycardia, more than 160 bpm. Fetal heart rate (FHR) monitoring may be done by electronic fetal monitoring (EFM) as well as auscultation or ultrasound with an abdominal transducer, but tracings can be poor with an active fetus, with maternal movement, and with hydramnios. Telemetry with ultrasound or fetal ECG transducers and external uterine pressure transducers can also be used to monitor FHR. This type of battery-operated monitoring can be used while the mother ambulates.

**12. A:** While the neonate's bilirubin is elevated (normal range 3.4 to 11.5 mg/dL at 1 to 2 days), only continued observation and jaundice assessment is indicated at this time. Physiologic hyperbilirubinemia is common in newborns and is usually benign, resulting from immature hepatic function and increased RBC hemolysis. Infants have larger red blood cells with a shorter life than adults, leading to more RBC destruction and resulting in an increased load of serum bilirubin, which the liver of the newborn cannot handle. Onset is usually within 24 to 48 hours, peaking in 72 hours for full-term or 5 days for preterm infants and declining within a week. Phototherapy is the indicated treatment for total serum bilirubin greater than or equal to 18 mg/dL for those at medium risk.

**13. D:** First stage: This stage signals onset of labor with regular contractions and proceeds until the cervix is fully dilated. There are 3 phases: latent, active, and transition. The latent phase may persist for 8.5 hours for nullipara and 5.3 hours for the multipara. The cervix begins to dilate (less than or equal to 3 cm) and contractions may occur every 3-30 minutes, lasting 20-40 seconds. The intensity of the contractions is usually mild to moderate (25-40 mm Hg per intrauterine pressure catheter [IUPC]). The mother is usually able to cope with discomfort and may feel some anxiety.

**14. C:** The head circumference is usually about 2 cm greater than the chest circumference, so the head circumference should be about 36 cm.

| | |
|---|---|
| Head | Disproportionately large for body |
| Body | Long with prominent abdomen and narrow hips |
| Extremities | Short and in flexed position; hands clenched<br>Feet are usually dorsiflexed after breech birth. |
| Neck | Short and chin resting on chest |
| Weight | 2500-4000 g (average about 3400)<br>Physiologic weight loss is 5-10% for full term and 15% for preterm. |
| Length | 45-55 cm (average 50 cm) |
| Head circumference | 32-38 cm (usually 2 cm greater than chest circumference) |
| Chest circumference | Chest rounded and 30-36 cm |

**15. C:** Palpate the thyroid gland from behind with patient's neck extended, noting enlargement and symmetry. Auscultate enlarged thyroid: Bruit may indicate hyperthyroidism. Inspect thyroid and cricoid cartilages and trachea, noting deviations from midline and asymmetrical spacing and observations during swallowing (all should elevate). Note swelling of parotid or submaxillary glands. Palpate lymph nodes with head slightly flexed (nodes should be moveable). Note any swelling or tenderness. Examine carotid artery and jugular veins and evaluate jugular venous pressure. Note pulse intensity and auscultate for bruit (indicating carotid obstruction).

**16. C:** A total score of 7 or higher out of a range of 0 to 10 is a sign of good health. APGAR is a quick evaluation of a newborn's physical condition, to determine if emergency medical care is needed and is administered 1 minute and 5 minutes after birth.

| Sign | 0 | 1 | 2 |
|---|---|---|---|
| Appearance (skin color) | Cyanotic or pallor over entire body | Normal, except for the extremities | Entire body normal |
| Pulse (heart rate) | Absent | Less than 100 bpm | Greater than 100 bpm |
| Grimace (reflex irritability) | Unresponsive | Grimace | Infant sneezes, coughs, and recoils |
| Activity (muscle tone) | Absent | Flexed limbs | Infant moves freely |
| Respiration (breathing rate and effort) | Absent | Bradypnea, dyspnea | Good breathing and crying |

**17. A:** Erythema toxicum is a skin eruption of erythematous papules, vesicles, and sometimes pustules. Erythema toxicum is essentially benign and occurs in more than 50% of newborns. It is a generalized rash everywhere except the palms and soles of the feet, usually occurring 2-3 days after birth. Neonatal pustular melanosis is a benign rash (vesicles and macules) but not associated with erythema. Cutis marmorata is a disorder in which the infant's skin mottles or marbles when exposed to cold, because the superficial blood vessels dilate and contract at the same time. Epidermolysis bullosa (EB) comprises genetic blistering disorders in which friction or trauma to the skin causes blisters to form.

**18. C:** Special precautions are indicated during delivery with shoulder dystocia. If meconium is noted, then the infant's nose and mouth should be suctioned before the infant's shoulders are delivered. There are four steps used to facilitate delivery. Do the McRoberts maneuver, in which the thighs are lifted and hyperflexed to elevate the pubic bone. Apply suprapubic pressure externally over the wedged shoulder while traction is continued. Manually rotate the infant's head and upper body while continuing suprapubic pressure. Finally, pull the posterior arm out of the birth canal, flex the elbow, and deliver the forearm over the chest wall.

**19. D:** The midwife should refer the woman to a specialist. Placenta previa occurs when the placenta implants over or near the internal cervical os. Implantation may be complete (covering the entire opening), partial, or marginal (to the edge of the cervical opening). Women with placenta previa have increased incidences of hemorrhage in the third trimester. Symptoms include painless bleeding after the 20$^{th}$ week of gestation. Diagnosis is per ultrasound. Vaginal examination with digit or speculum should be avoided. The condition may correct itself as the uterus expands, but bed rest may be needed. Emergency C-section is done for uncontrolled bleeding.

**20. B:** Intravenous acyclovir is given to infants exposed to herpes virus. Most vertical transmissions occur when the neonate travels through a colonized birth canal. The transmission rate from women with a primary HSV infection is approximately 50%, while the transmission rate is 1-2% if the infection is a recurrence of HSV. Signs of a neonatal infection with HSV include the following:

- Skin, eye, and mucous membrane may blister at 10-12 days of life.
- Disseminated disease may spread to multiple organs, leading to pneumonitis, hepatitis, and intravascular coagulation.
- Encephalitis may be the only presentation, with signs of lethargy, irritability, poor feeding, and seizures.

**21. B:** The scalp stimulation test (SST) is a noninvasive method of assessing fetal status (as opposed to fetal scalp blood testing). If the fetus is not under distress, then a normal response is an increase in heart rate by 15 bpm for at least 15 seconds. Reactivity is associated with well-being of the fetus, but failure to react does not provide definitive evidence of compromise and must be confirmed by other measures. SST is conducted by applying firm pressure with the examining finger on the fetal scalp.

**22. C:** The uterine fundus (curvature at the top) can be palpated above the symphysis pubis by about 10 to 12 weeks' gestation, and fundal height can be used to estimate duration of gestation and growth of the fetus. Starting at about 16 weeks' gestation and lasting until week 36, the fundal height (from top of symphysis pubis to top of fundus, measured in centimeters) usually conforms with the weeks of gestation, so 18 cm is consistent with 18 weeks' gestation in a pregnancy with a normal single fetus. At 20 weeks (20 cm), the fundus is usually at the umbilicus.

**23. D:** Dissociation relaxation teaches the mother to tighten just one set of voluntary muscles and relax the rest (neuromuscular dissociation) to prepare her to relax all voluntary muscles during uterine contractions. This technique uses discomfort to help the mother dissociate from the pain.

For example, the partner may grasp the upper arms and rotate the skin outward to create a burning sensation. Then, the woman relaxes other muscles in a sequence of contracting, holding, and relaxing. The usual sequence is right arm, left arm, right leg, left leg, both arms, both legs, right arm and leg, and finally left arm and leg.

**24. B:** The first trimester can be considered a time of psychosocial crisis. The woman can experience a period of stress and anxiety, which can have a profound impact on her relationship with her partner or husband. Fears of miscarriage are not unusual. The midwife should provide factual information and reassurance. These concerns by the mother can be minimized by her partner's involvement in the pregnancy, such as by accompanying her to Lamaze classes and prenatal visits.

**25. A:** Energy needs of the mother usually remain stable during the first trimester but an added 300 kilocalories a day are needed during the second and third trimester for a singleton and 600 kilocalories a day for twins. Generally, a pregnant woman requires about 60 g of protein daily and 4 to 5 cups of milk (or equivalent). Diet should include 2 to 4 servings of fruit and 3 to 5 servings of vegetables. Simple carbohydrates (sugar, flour) should be limited and replaced by whole grains, which are high in B vitamins. Fat should constitute about 30% of total caloric intake.

**26. D:** The designated landmark for breech presentations is the sacrum (S), for vertex presentations the occiput (O), for face presentations the mentum (M), and for shoulder presentations the acromion process (A). Fetal position is determined by the relationship of the presenting fetal part (designated landmark) to the maternal pelvis. When describing position, three different notations are required:

- Right or left (R or L) side of maternal pelvis
- Landmark designation (S, O, M, or A)
- Position of landmark in relation to pelvis: anterior (A), posterior (P) or transverse (T)

**27. B:** Tongue extrusion is elicited by touching the tip of the tongue. A normal response is for the neonate to push the tongue out of the mouth. Continuous or repetitive extrusion indicates CNS abnormalities or seizure activity. The tongue is examined for ridge of frenulum tissue on underside (tongue-tied, although this is not clipped) and evidence of protrusion or hypertrophy, which can indicate various disorders (such as Down syndrome and hypothyroidism). Bluish swelling of the frenulum may indicate mucous/salivary gland retention cyst.

**28. A:**

| | |
|---|---|
| Weight | 2500-4000 g (average about 3400)<br>Physiologic weight loss is 5-10% for full term and 15% for preterm. |
| Length | 45-55 cm (average 50 cm) |
| Head circumference | 32-38 cm (usually 2 cm greater than chest circumference) |
| Chest circumference | 30-36 cm |
| Temperature | Temperature drops rapidly (skin temperature falls 0.3°C/minute) after birth with exposure to ambient room temperature but stabilizes within 8-12 hours. Temperature is usually measured by axillary method (for 3 minutes) and ranges from 36.3°C to 37.0°C. |
| Blood pressure | 56-77/33-50 mm Hg |
| Pulse | 120-120 bpm awake; 100 bpm asleep; 180 bmp crying |

| | |
|---|---|
| Respiration | 30-60 per minute |

**29. C:** Asian, African American, and other dark-skinned infants may have Mongolian spots (blue-black discoloration) on the buttocks and dorsal area. *Nevus flammeus* (port-wine stain) is a demarcated unraised red-purple lesion caused by capillaries below the epidermis. *Nevus vasculosus* (strawberry mark) is a capillary hemangioma and is a raised, demarcated dark red lesion. Mottling, or irregular discoloration, is common for hours to weeks after birth and may relate to prolonged periods of apnea or chilling.

**30. C:**

| Reflex | Eliciting reflex | Normal response |
|---|---|---|
| **Moro (startle)** | Make a loud sound or give the infant a gentle jolt. | The infant extends the arms, legs, and neck, and then pulls back the arms and legs. The infant may also cry. |
| **Palmar Grasping** | Stroke the infant's palm. | The infant responds by grasping the finger. |
| **Rooting** | Stroke the side of the infant's cheek. | The infant turns the head in the same direction as the touch, and opens their mouth to feed. |
| **Sucking** | Touch the infant's mouth. | The infant sucks. |

**31. A:** Hypertension present before 20 weeks' gestation or beyond 6 weeks postpartum is most often related to chronic hypertension, which puts the patient at increased risk of developing preeclampsia, so the patient must be monitored carefully. Preeclampsia is hypertension with proteinuria, usually occurring in the second half of gestation. While edema usually occurs with preeclampsia, it is also a common finding in pregnancy. Severe preeclampsia is BP greater than 160-180/110 and proteinuria greater than 1 g with 24-hour urine collection or more than 2 g with dipstick.

**32. D:** *Neisseria gonorrhoeae* infections may result in recurrent infection, pelvic inflammatory disease (PID), chronic pain, and infertility. Women who become pregnant and have a history of gonorrhea with salpingitis are 7 to 10 times more likely to have an ectopic pregnancy. Signs of infection (dysuria and green foul-smelling discharge from the urethra and the vagina) may occur 3 to 5 days after contact. However, many women are asymptomatic, especially on initial infection. Vaginal delivery increases neonatal risk and can result in severe conjunctivitis, rupture of the globe, and blindness; however, routine prophylaxis (usually erythromycin ointment) to the neonate's eyes is effective.

**33. B:** The woman should be advised to limit weight gain to 15 pounds. Infants of obese and morbidly obese women are often macrosomic (large) and may suffer fetal distress, early neonatal death, meconium aspiration, shoulder dystocia, and/or complications from Cesarean birth. Recommended weight gains:

- Underweight: 28-40 lbs
- Normal weight: 25-35 lbs
- Overweight: 15-25 lbs
- Obese: 15 lbs

The mother must maintain an adequate nutritional diet. Maternal malnutrition can have a profound effect on the developing fetus. If malnutrition occurs during the stages of cell division, then cells may not divide properly, causing permanent damage.

**34. A:** A woman with one previous Cesarean section and a low transverse uterine incision is the best candidate for vaginal birth. A woman with 2 or more previous Cesarean sections may attempt vaginal births. In all cases, a physician, an anesthesiologist, and adequate staff must be present and available throughout labor to provide a Cesarean section if necessary. Contraindications to attempting vaginal delivery include a T or classic incision, history of myomectomy, contracted pelvis, obstetrical complications precluding vaginal birth, and inadequate facilities or staff to provide emergency Cesarean section if it is needed.

**35. B:** Backache during pregnancy can result from increased hormone levels causing softening of cartilage and increased lumbosacral curvature. Muscle strain, fatigues, poor body mechanics, and carrying twins all contribute to backache. Management includes the following measures:

- Do the pelvic-tilt exercise and begin modified exercise program, such as swimming, beginning with stretching.
- Utilize correct body mechanics and avoid heavy lifting, reaching for things on high surfaces, and wearing high-heeled shoes.
- Adjust height of work surfaces.
- Apply heat to lower back.
- Use back support in chair/bed and stand straight and avoid slumping.

**36. D:**

| Symmetric IUGR | Asymmetric IUGR |
|---|---|
| Both head and body are small (growth-restricted). | Large head in proportion to the body; the head is spared. |
| Occurs early in pregnancy. | The head is normal in size for gestational age, while the body is growth-restricted. |
| Common causes are chromosomal abnormalities, chronic hypertension, infections, substance abuse, and severe malnutrition. | Occurs late in pregnancy. |
| | Common causes include placental insufficiency, preeclampsia, and poor weight gain. |

**37. A:** This is normal lochia rubra:

| | | |
|---|---|---|
| Rubra | Days 1 to 3 or 4 | Dark red discharge, containing epithelial cells, red and white blood cells, bacteria, decidua shreds, lanugo, vernix caseosa, and sometimes meconium. Clots should not exceed nickel size, as large clots may indicate hemorrhage or bleeding from vaginal lacerations. |
| Serosa | Days 4 to 10 | Pinkish to brownish discharge, containing serous exudate, decidua shreds, red and white blood cells, cervical mucus, and various microorganisms. |
| Alba | Additional 2 to 85 days (average 24) | Yellowish discharge contains primarily white blood cells, epithelial cells, decidual cells, fat, mucus, and bacteria. The cervix is closed when lochia alba flow stops, so the danger of infection ceases. |

**38. C:** Mastitis causes induration, swelling, erythema, increasing fever, acute pain, and sometimes painful abscesses. The infected area may be localized or generalized. The mother may have chills and flu-like symptoms before obvious inflammation of the breast. Usually the mother becomes infected from the infant (generally *Staphylococcus aureus)* so breastfeeding does not endanger the neonate. Treatment includes antibiotics (usually penicillin G, dicloxacillin, or erythromycin) and nursing (or pumping or expressing) on the affected side to prevent abscess formation. Applying heat or massaging the breasts in a warm shower may increase circulation. Pain relief includes alternating warm and cold compresses and acetaminophen or ibuprofen.

**39. B:** These are signs of postpartum depression, so the nurse should make a referral for a psychiatric consult. Onset may occur any time within the first year, but is most common around week 4 postpartum, before the onset of menses. Duration varies but is usually 3 to 14 months (half symptomatic at 6 months). Symptoms are typical of depression. The mother may be irritable and hostile, especially toward the child. She may also be suicidal. Treatment may include psychotherapy, antidepressants, antipsychotics, and/or lithium. In some cases, the child may need to be cared for by others until the mother's depression lessens.

**40. D:** The mother should increase nursing frequency to every 2 to 3 hours, nursing until tissue softens. If the areola is taut, some milk should be manually expressed before the baby latches on. Breast pumping may make engorgement worse but may be used briefly to soften the areola. Cold compresses applied to the breasts after nursing may relieve discomfort. Engorgement almost always recedes in 24 to 48 hours, so the nurse should encourage the mother to continue breastfeeding.

**41. A:** Café au lait spots (CAL) are flat skin lesions with increased melanin content and regular or irregular borders. If the CAL spots are faint, one can use a Wood lamp to make them easier to see. Fewer than 3 café au lait spots have no clinical significance. However, 6 or more café au lait spots with a diameter larger than 5 mm occur in 95% of patients with neurofibromatosis type 1 (NF1), a disorder of chromosome 17. Lisch nodules on the child's iris and Crowe's sign (freckles on the axilla and inguinal area) corroborate the diagnosis of NF1.

**42. C:** Sunscreen products are usually safe for pregnant women, who often experience an increase in acne because of hormonal changes but should avoid cleansing preparations that contain salicylic acid or anti-aging compounds with retinoids. Women should avoid hair dye and permanent waves because some of the chemicals are teratogenic, especially during the first trimester. Henna is a natural product that is safe. Lemon juice can be used to lighten facial hair rather than bleach products. Soy products may increase melasma because of estrogenic properties. Chemical hair removers and sunscreen products are generally safe for pregnant women.

**43. A:** While all of these are important, the initial action should be to determine the status of the cervical dilation and effacement. With any indication of membrane rupture, the examination should be done with a speculum rather than a digital exam, which may increase the risk of infection. Palpation should be used to determine the strength, duration, and frequency of contractions. A urine specimen should be obtained because urinary infections may cause premature contractions. An ultrasound is used to determine the fetal gestational age. Tocolytics may be used if labor persists.

**44. B:** The most common neonatal injury associated with macrosomia is shoulder dystocia. Traumatic brain injury and brachial plexus injury are less common but may occur. Fetal macrosomia, an exceptionally large fetus, poses problems for vaginal delivery because of the size of the infant. Fetal macrosomia is defined variably as greater than the $90^{th}$ percentile for weight according to gestational age or greater than 4500 g. Fundal height greater than 4 cm above what is expected for gestational age may be an indication. Fetal macrosomia is common with infants of diabetic mothers, as well as obese mothers or those who gain an excessive amount of weight during pregnancy.

**45. D:** Kitzinger encourages women to take an active part in the natural birthing process and encourages alternatives to the usual hospital birthing procedures, including home births, birth rooms, and water births. Bradley encourages natural childbirth and begins with a focus on the woman's health, including avoiding risk factors, ensuring good nutrition, and learning to handle pain. Lamaze encourages women to take control of their bodies and utilizes various techniques (dissociation relaxation, relaxation exercises, and breathing patterns) to alleviate discomfort and facilitate birth. HypnoBirthing combines natural birthing and self-hypnosis to help the mother eliminate stress and fear related to birthing.

**46. C:** A woman with mild preeclampsia is usually treated initially with bed rest, in the left lateral decubitus position as much as possible since this maximizes cardiac output and blood flow to the uterus and helps to normalize blood pressure. The woman should be weighed daily and monitored carefully. If symptoms worsen, then magnesium sulfate and antihypertensives may be indicated, as well as anticonvulsants to prevent seizures. Labor may be induced or a Cesarean done, especially if there is maternal or fetal distress.

**47. C:** A woman should be encouraged to respond to her own urge to push rather than instructed to hold her breath to slow birthing, because this can result in excess stretching of the perineum and decreased blood flow. The lithotomy and other recumbent positions are used for the convenience of medical personnel but are not natural positions for delivery and can also result in excess stretching of the perineum. Unless there is maternal or fetal distress, the second stage of labor should be allowed to progress at its own speed.

**48. B:** If signs of placental separation are evident and the fundus is firm, then the midwife may apply gentle traction to the cord while applying pressure on the fundus to encourage expulsion. Signs of placental separation usually occur between 5 and 30 minutes after birth. These signs include:

- Globular-shaped uterus
- Fundus rising in the abdomen
- Increased gush or trickling of blood
- Umbilical cord protruding further from the vagina

A placenta is considered retained if it has not separated in over 30 minutes after delivery.

**49. C:** The midwife should continue to apply pressure to the presenting part while the mother elevates her knees to her chest until Cesarean. A prolapse of the umbilical cord occurs when the umbilical cord precedes the fetus in the birth canal and becomes entrapped by the descending fetus. As contractions occur and the head descends, pressure is applied to the umbilical cord, occluding blood flow and causing hypoxia and bradycardia. The decrease in blood flow through the umbilical vessels can cause impaired gas exchange, and if pressure on the cord is not relieved, the fetus can suffer severe neurological damage or death.

**50. D:** Rhinorrhea, nasal irritation, and perforation of the septum are consistent with intranasal use of cocaine or amphetamines. Maternal cocaine use increases the risk of premature birth and causes serious consequences for the neonate after birth, including cerebral infarctions, nonduodenal intestinal atresia, anal atresia, NEC, defects of the limbs, and genitourinary defects. Maternal use of amphetamines causes hypertension and tachycardia, which can cause miscarriage, abruptio placentae, and premature delivery. Vasoconstriction affects placental vessels, decreasing circulation, nutrition, and oxygen to the fetus. Methamphetamines can cross the placental barrier and cause fetal hypertension and prenatal strokes and damage to the heart and other organs.

# How to Overcome Test Anxiety

Just the thought of taking a test is enough to make most people a little nervous. A test is an important event that can have a long-term impact on your future, so it's important to take it seriously and it's natural to feel anxious about performing well. But just because anxiety is normal, that doesn't mean that it's helpful in test taking, or that you should simply accept it as part of your life. Anxiety can have a variety of effects. These effects can be mild, like making you feel slightly nervous, or severe, like blocking your ability to focus or remember even a simple detail.

If you experience test anxiety—whether severe or mild—it's important to know how to beat it. To discover this, first you need to understand what causes test anxiety.

## Causes of Test Anxiety

While we often think of anxiety as an uncontrollable emotional state, it can actually be caused by simple, practical things. One of the most common causes of test anxiety is that a person does not feel adequately prepared for their test. This feeling can be the result of many different issues such as poor study habits or lack of organization, but the most common culprit is time management. Starting to study too late, failing to organize your study time to cover all of the material, or being distracted while you study will mean that you're not well prepared for the test. This may lead to cramming the night before, which will cause you to be physically and mentally exhausted for the test. Poor time management also contributes to feelings of stress, fear, and hopelessness as you realize you are not well prepared but don't know what to do about it.

Other times, test anxiety is not related to your preparation for the test but comes from unresolved fear. This may be a past failure on a test, or poor performance on tests in general. It may come from comparing yourself to others who seem to be performing better or from the stress of living up to expectations. Anxiety may be driven by fears of the future—how failure on this test would affect your educational and career goals. These fears are often completely irrational, but they can still negatively impact your test performance.

## Elements of Test Anxiety

As mentioned earlier, test anxiety is considered to be an emotional state, but it has physical and mental components as well. Sometimes you may not even realize that you are suffering from test anxiety until you notice the physical symptoms. These can include trembling hands, rapid heartbeat, sweating, nausea, and tense muscles. Extreme anxiety may lead to fainting or vomiting. Obviously, any of these symptoms can have a negative impact on testing. It is important to recognize them as soon as they begin to occur so that you can address the problem before it damages your performance.

The mental components of test anxiety include trouble focusing and inability to remember learned information. During a test, your mind is on high alert, which can help you recall information and stay focused for an extended period of time. However, anxiety interferes with your mind's natural processes, causing you to blank out, even on the questions you know well. The strain of testing during anxiety makes it difficult to stay focused, especially on a test that may take several hours. Extreme anxiety can take a huge mental toll, making it difficult not only to recall test information but even to understand the test questions or pull your thoughts together.

## Effects of Test Anxiety

Test anxiety is like a disease—if left untreated, it will get progressively worse. Anxiety leads to poor performance, and this reinforces the feelings of fear and failure, which in turn lead to poor performances on subsequent tests. It can grow from a mild nervousness to a crippling condition. If allowed to progress, test anxiety can have a big impact on your schooling, and consequently on your future.

Test anxiety can spread to other parts of your life. Anxiety on tests can become anxiety in any stressful situation, and blanking on a test can turn into panicking in a job situation. But fortunately, you don't have to let anxiety rule your testing and determine your grades. There are a number of relatively simple steps you can take to move past anxiety and function normally on a test and in the rest of life.

## Physical Steps for Beating Test Anxiety

While test anxiety is a serious problem, the good news is that it can be overcome. It doesn't have to control your ability to think and remember information. While it may take time, you can begin taking steps today to beat anxiety.

Just as your first hint that you may be struggling with anxiety comes from the physical symptoms, the first step to treating it is also physical. Rest is crucial for having a clear, strong mind. If you are tired, it is much easier to give in to anxiety. But if you establish good sleep habits, your body and mind will be ready to perform optimally, without the strain of exhaustion. Additionally, sleeping well helps you to retain information better, so you're more likely to recall the answers when you see the test questions.

Getting good sleep means more than going to bed on time. It's important to allow your brain time to relax. Take study breaks from time to time so it doesn't get overworked, and don't study right before bed. Take time to rest your mind before trying to rest your body, or you may find it difficult to fall asleep.

Along with sleep, other aspects of physical health are important in preparing for a test. Good nutrition is vital for good brain function. Sugary foods and drinks may give a burst of energy but this burst is followed by a crash, both physically and emotionally. Instead, fuel your body with protein and vitamin-rich foods.

Also, drink plenty of water. Dehydration can lead to headaches and exhaustion, especially if your brain is already under stress from the rigors of the test. Particularly if your test is a long one, drink water during the breaks. And if possible, take an energy-boosting snack to eat between sections.

Along with sleep and diet, a third important part of physical health is exercise. Maintaining a steady workout schedule is helpful, but even taking 5-minute study breaks to walk can help get your blood pumping faster and clear your head. Exercise also releases endorphins, which contribute to a positive feeling and can help combat test anxiety.

When you nurture your physical health, you are also contributing to your mental health. If your body is healthy, your mind is much more likely to be healthy as well. So take time to rest, nourish your body with healthy food and water, and get moving as much as possible. Taking these physical steps will make you stronger and more able to take the mental steps necessary to overcome test anxiety.

## Mental Steps for Beating Test Anxiety

Working on the mental side of test anxiety can be more challenging, but as with the physical side, there are clear steps you can take to overcome it. As mentioned earlier, test anxiety often stems from lack of preparation, so the obvious solution is to prepare for the test. Effective studying may be the most important weapon you have for beating test anxiety, but you can and should employ several other mental tools to combat fear.

First, boost your confidence by reminding yourself of past success—tests or projects that you aced. If you're putting as much effort into preparing for this test as you did for those, there's no reason you should expect to fail here. Work hard to prepare; then trust your preparation.

Second, surround yourself with encouraging people. It can be helpful to find a study group, but be sure that the people you're around will encourage a positive attitude. If you spend time with others who are anxious or cynical, this will only contribute to your own anxiety. Look for others who are motivated to study hard from a desire to succeed, not from a fear of failure.

Third, reward yourself. A test is physically and mentally tiring, even without anxiety, and it can be helpful to have something to look forward to. Plan an activity following the test, regardless of the outcome, such as going to a movie or getting ice cream.

When you are taking the test, if you find yourself beginning to feel anxious, remind yourself that you know the material. Visualize successfully completing the test. Then take a few deep, relaxing breaths and return to it. Work through the questions carefully but with confidence, knowing that you are capable of succeeding.

Developing a healthy mental approach to test taking will also aid in other areas of life. Test anxiety affects more than just the actual test—it can be damaging to your mental health and even contribute to depression. It's important to beat test anxiety before it becomes a problem for more than testing.

## Study Strategy

Being prepared for the test is necessary to combat anxiety, but what does being prepared look like? You may study for hours on end and still not feel prepared. What you need is a strategy for test prep. The next few pages outline our recommended steps to help you plan out and conquer the challenge of preparation.

### Step 1: Scope Out the Test

Learn everything you can about the format (multiple choice, essay, etc.) and what will be on the test. Gather any study materials, course outlines, or sample exams that may be available. Not only will this help you to prepare, but knowing what to expect can help to alleviate test anxiety.

### Step 2: Map Out the Material

Look through the textbook or study guide and make note of how many chapters or sections it has. Then divide these over the time you have. For example, if a book has 15 chapters and you have five days to study, you need to cover three chapters each day. Even better, if you have the time, leave an extra day at the end for overall review after you have gone through the material in depth.

If time is limited, you may need to prioritize the material. Look through it and make note of which sections you think you already have a good grasp on, and which need review. While you are studying, skim quickly through the familiar sections and take more time on the challenging parts.

Write out your plan so you don't get lost as you go. Having a written plan also helps you feel more in control of the study, so anxiety is less likely to arise from feeling overwhelmed at the amount to cover.

### Step 3: Gather Your Tools

Decide what study method works best for you. Do you prefer to highlight in the book as you study and then go back over the highlighted portions? Or do you type out notes of the important information? Or is it helpful to make flashcards that you can carry with you? Assemble the pens, index cards, highlighters, post-it notes, and any other materials you may need so you won't be distracted by getting up to find things while you study.

If you're having a hard time retaining the information or organizing your notes, experiment with different methods. For example, try color-coding by subject with colored pens, highlighters, or post-it notes. If you learn better by hearing, try recording yourself reading your notes so you can listen while in the car, working out, or simply sitting at your desk. Ask a friend to quiz you from your flashcards, or try teaching someone the material to solidify it in your mind.

### Step 4: Create Your Environment

It's important to avoid distractions while you study. This includes both the obvious distractions like visitors and the subtle distractions like an uncomfortable chair (or a too-comfortable couch that makes you want to fall asleep). Set up the best study environment possible: good lighting and a comfortable work area. If background music helps you focus, you may want to turn it on, but otherwise keep the room quiet. If you are using a computer to take notes, be sure you don't have any other windows open, especially applications like social media, games, or anything else that could distract you. Silence your phone and turn off notifications. Be sure to keep water close by so you stay hydrated while you study (but avoid unhealthy drinks and snacks).

Also, take into account the best time of day to study. Are you freshest first thing in the morning? Try to set aside some time then to work through the material. Is your mind clearer in the afternoon or evening? Schedule your study session then. Another method is to study at the same time of day that you will take the test, so that your brain gets used to working on the material at that time and will be ready to focus at test time.

### Step 5: Study!

Once you have done all the study preparation, it's time to settle into the actual studying. Sit down, take a few moments to settle your mind so you can focus, and begin to follow your study plan. Don't give in to distractions or let yourself procrastinate. This is your time to prepare so you'll be ready to fearlessly approach the test. Make the most of the time and stay focused.

Of course, you don't want to burn out. If you study too long you may find that you're not retaining the information very well. Take regular study breaks. For example, taking five minutes out of every hour to walk briskly, breathing deeply and swinging your arms, can help your mind stay fresh.

As you get to the end of each chapter or section, it's a good idea to do a quick review. Remind yourself of what you learned and work on any difficult parts. When you feel that you've mastered the material, move on to the next part. At the end of your study session, briefly skim through your notes again.

But while review is helpful, cramming last minute is NOT. If at all possible, work ahead so that you won't need to fit all your study into the last day. Cramming overloads your brain with more information than it can process and retain, and your tired mind may struggle to recall even previously learned information when it is overwhelmed with last-minute study. Also, the urgent nature of cramming and the stress placed on your brain contribute to anxiety. You'll be more likely to go to the test feeling unprepared and having trouble thinking clearly.

So don't cram, and don't stay up late before the test, even just to review your notes at a leisurely pace. Your brain needs rest more than it needs to go over the information again. In fact, plan to finish your studies by noon or early afternoon the day before the test. Give your brain the rest of the day to relax or focus on other things, and get a good night's sleep. Then you will be fresh for the test and better able to recall what you've studied.

### Step 6: Take a Practice Test

Many courses offer sample tests, either online or in the study materials. This is an excellent resource to check whether you have mastered the material, as well as to prepare for the test format and environment.

Check the test format ahead of time: the number of questions, the type (multiple choice, free response, etc.), and the time limit. Then create a plan for working through them. For example, if you have 30 minutes to take a 60-question test, your limit is 30 seconds per question. Spend less time on the questions you know well so that you can take more time on the difficult ones.

If you have time to take several practice tests, take the first one open book, with no time limit. Work through the questions at your own pace and make sure you fully understand them. Gradually work up to taking a test under test conditions: sit at a desk with all study materials put away and set a timer. Pace yourself to make sure you finish the test with time to spare and go back to check your answers if you have time.

After each test, check your answers. On the questions you missed, be sure you understand why you missed them. Did you misread the question (tests can use tricky wording)? Did you forget the information? Or was it something you hadn't learned? Go back and study any shaky areas that the practice tests reveal.

Taking these tests not only helps with your grade, but also aids in combating test anxiety. If you're already used to the test conditions, you're less likely to worry about it, and working through tests until you're scoring well gives you a confidence boost. Go through the practice tests until you feel comfortable, and then you can go into the test knowing that you're ready for it.

## Test Tips

On test day, you should be confident, knowing that you've prepared well and are ready to answer the questions. But aside from preparation, there are several test day strategies you can employ to maximize your performance.

First, as stated before, get a good night's sleep the night before the test (and for several nights before that, if possible). Go into the test with a fresh, alert mind rather than staying up late to study.

Try not to change too much about your normal routine on the day of the test. It's important to eat a nutritious breakfast, but if you normally don't eat breakfast at all, consider eating just a protein bar. If you're a coffee drinker, go ahead and have your normal coffee. Just make sure you time it so that the caffeine doesn't wear off right in the middle of your test. Avoid sugary beverages, and drink enough water to stay hydrated but not so much that you need a restroom break 10 minutes into the test. If your test isn't first thing in the morning, consider going for a walk or doing a light workout before the test to get your blood flowing.

Allow yourself enough time to get ready, and leave for the test with plenty of time to spare so you won't have the anxiety of scrambling to arrive in time. Another reason to be early is to select a good seat. It's helpful to sit away from doors and windows, which can be distracting. Find a good seat, get out your supplies, and settle your mind before the test begins.

When the test begins, start by going over the instructions carefully, even if you already know what to expect. Make sure you avoid any careless mistakes by following the directions.

Then begin working through the questions, pacing yourself as you've practiced. If you're not sure on an answer, don't spend too much time on it, and don't let it shake your confidence. Either skip it and come back later, or eliminate as many wrong answers as possible and guess among the remaining ones. Don't dwell on these questions as you continue—put them out of your mind and focus on what lies ahead.

Be sure to read all of the answer choices, even if you're sure the first one is the right answer. Sometimes you'll find a better one if you keep reading. But don't second-guess yourself if you do immediately know the answer. Your gut instinct is usually right. Don't let test anxiety rob you of the information you know.

If you have time at the end of the test (and if the test format allows), go back and review your answers. Be cautious about changing any, since your first instinct tends to be correct, but make sure you didn't misread any of the questions or accidentally mark the wrong answer choice. Look over any you skipped and make an educated guess.

At the end, leave the test feeling confident. You've done your best, so don't waste time worrying about your performance or wishing you could change anything. Instead, celebrate the successful completion of this test. And finally, use this test to learn how to deal with anxiety even better next time.

**Review Video: Test Anxiety**
Visit mometrix.com/academy and enter code: 100340

## Important Qualification

Not all anxiety is created equal. If your test anxiety is causing major issues in your life beyond the classroom or testing center, or if you are experiencing troubling physical symptoms related to your anxiety, it may be a sign of a serious physiological or psychological condition. If this sounds like your situation, we strongly encourage you to seek professional help.

## Online Resources

Due to our efforts to try to keep this book to a manageable length, we've created a link that will give you access to all of your online resources:

**mometrix.com/resources719/midwives**

# It's Your Moment, Let's Celebrate It!

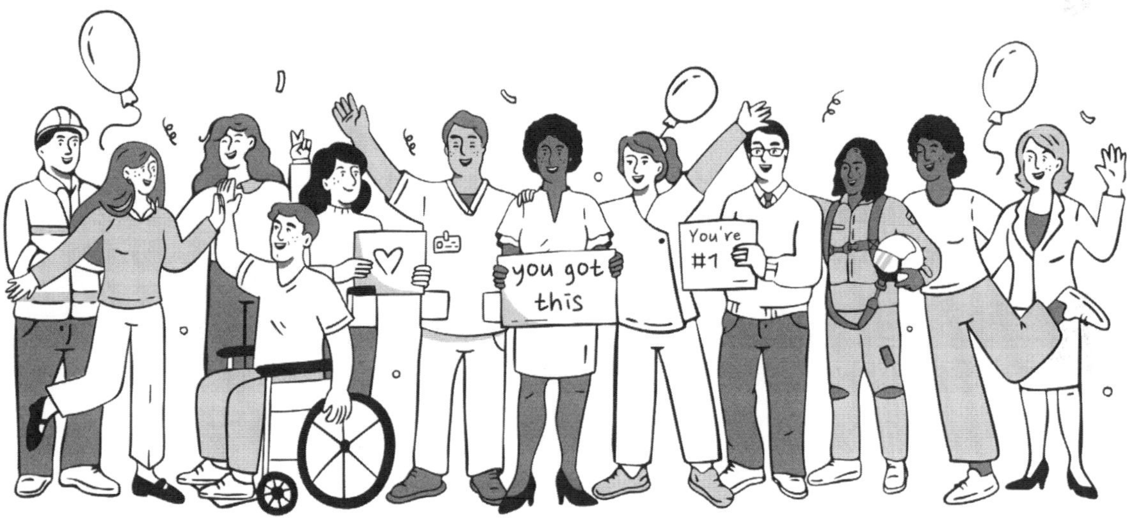


**Share your story @mometrixtestpreparation**